GUT

How to feed and protect your Second Brain to improve your health

Malik Johnson

© Copyright 2015 by

TABLE OF CONTENTS

INTRODUCTION

For individuals who are occupied with finding out about the gut and how to protect it, strolling into a large bookshop can be as confounding as looking for "GUT- How to feed and protect your Second Brain" books at amazon.com. At first, there seems, by all accounts, to be an unending determination to browse. Most vast bookshops have a few racks committed to Second Brain. They incorporate books on The Gut – Our Second Brain, Second Brain and the Chemistry of Addiction, Stomach ulcers and why they come to be and Natural remedies for Stomach Ulcer, Stomach Ulcer treatment, what's more, obviously, The Gut. On the other hand, even the Gut books appear to shift away from the main topic to other topics. Different books concentrate on the Gut as a specific subject, so they do not have an expansive picture. This book is expected to address these issues. It is intended to be a solitary beginning point for anybody keen on the points of the gut, or the second brain. The book will surely cover particular problems and issues regarding the stomach and how they depend on each other to be effective.

CHAPTER ONE:
THE GUT – OUR SECOND BRAIN

What exactly is the Second Brain?

The gut has its own sensory system known as the "enteric sensory system." It is indispensably important to the operation of the human body and it even operates without information from the spinal code or the brain. The gut assumes a fundamental part in our passionate and physical prosperity. The sentiment "butterflies" in your stomach when you are anxious or energized or a sinking feeling in your gut when you fear something is your gut's method for speaking with you.

How is the Second Brain Different from the Brain in our Head?

The "second brain" or stomach brain is entirely different from the brain in our heads. Our cranial brain performs complex psychological capacities, for example, thinking, computations and making arrangements in view of rationale. Conversely, our second brain is natural and gets flags and messages with respect to our bodies and the environment that it sends back to our cranial brain and the other way around. Understanding the second brain and its capacities is the response to helping individuals who are pained with gastrointestinal issues that are frequently released by customary medicinal experts that regularly mark patients as hypochondriac.

Why is the Gut Called a Brain?

The second brain creates a tremendous quantity of mixtures including each kind of neurotransmitter found in the cranial brain. Truth be told, the gut (second brain) creates 95% of the compound serotonin. Without sufficient levels of serotonin, we experience sleeping disorders and depression.

How the Two Brains are connected?

The cranial and stomach brains are connected by a link known as the vagus nerve. Neurotransmission permits the two brains to have the capacity to speak with one another and to cooperate so that the body can work in congruity. At the point when these two brains interface - we have the capacity to coordinate, especially with ourselves. The second brain shapes and structures our passionate condition of being. The state of the belly causes feelings of dejection or energy, bitterness or happiness, and misery or satisfaction. In our gut lives the greater part of our enthusiastic impressions for the duration of our lives! Shielded from our mindfulness this tissue holds a number of our most important inner thoughts. Ultimately, the state of our inner thoughts manifests themselves physically.

These side effects behave like notice signs. It's our body's method for saying, "Pay attention to me! Pay attention to my gut!" With regard to the gut and our emotional Problems, analysts are starting to comprehend the intricate relationship between the second brain and mental issues. Specialists are finding out that depression, fractious gut disorder, ulcers, Parkinson's and Alzheimer's illnesses manifest at the level of both the brain and the gut. These diseases stay in a dormant yet highly sensitive state in most of the body's operational systems. This is in spite of the fact they may have entered the system many years prior to actual symptoms become visible.

Mend the Second Brain and the Rest will follow

Ten years back, I was encountering overwhelming feelings of tension and apprehension. I was additionally stuck in my inventive work. I attempted various mending methodologies under the sun without much success. In the process of mending, I discovered that the Taoists have known for quite a long time that the mid-region, and the feelings and strains inside it, are the reason for some infirmities and infections. I was fascinated.

A New Hope for Healing

The stagnant examples and apprehension of progress we hold inside ourselves prevent the blossoming of our potential. With the developing understanding of our second brain - unrest in mending is occurring. With the knowledge of the brain in our gut; its energy and capacity, we now have a chance to mend at the most profound level, to discover the meaning of our lives and to do our part in making the world we desire to see. We' vet all done it. Towards the beginning of another year we make resolutions. We are certain we most likely need to change yet converting our resolutions into practice is usually difficult. For instance, a companion might state that he is resolved to change an angle in his life. However, you may observe him and realize that in practical terms, he is not doing as he had indicated. How would you know?

Given that you realized that he was talking from his brain and not from his heart, such knowledge is important in agreeing or disagreeing with his opinions. However, it is when the heart is involved that we are able to change things concerning our whole lives. Eastern conventions and a small part of elusive western customs believe that a genuine heart is nurtured by good coordination between the brain and the stomach and is situated in the middle area around our stomach. Some researchers have found this to be the area around the kidney and some areas below the navel.

If you take a look at a person closely, it is possible to see where their focal point is offset. You may notice that their focal point of balance is in their shoulders or their head. This is not the best place. Having our focal point anywhere else apart from the sun-oriented plexus and Dan tien is not a good thing. It does not help in our focus either on the physical or emotional level.

Each neurotransmitter found in the brain can be found in the intestinal tract. The sunlight-based plexus is a system of nerve strands of the sensory system. It is made out of dark and white nerve substance or brain matter. The neurotransmitter, Serotonin, which is generally found in the intestinal tract, has been discovered to be inadequate in numerous individuals. This may lead to ill effects such as the feeling of wretchedness. It is the focal point of balance, wellbeing and instinct. Fundamentally, when we need to change viewpoints throughout our life, unfortunate propensities, negative feelings or when we need to grow new aptitudes or skills, say ice skating or tennis, it is important to communicate with our inner functions.

Paula, a companion of mine let me know that on the first occasion when she was included in an auto collision, her heart rate increased dramatically, her vitality was unsettled and she was stunned. This experience pushed her to go to attend chi gung classes. She learnt how to keep up her focal point of offset lower to the mid-section. Unbelievably, she was involved in another deadly accident with her car a year later. This time however, the chi gung classes, which taught her how to change her focal point lower to the mid-section, finally paid off. She found herself able to resist the urge to panic. The rhythm of her heart was more natural, her breathing smoother and she was more aware of everything going ahead around her.

Our digestion system, assimilation, development, and recuperating all happens in the system of plexus' beneath the waist. It all happens intuitively. This 'second brain' is the spot where change is made.

What Is Gut Health?

Your gut assumes a noteworthy part in your safety and wellbeing. Some 80-85% of your insusceptible cells are situated inside of your digestive framework. Your gut is an immense biological system of a trillion microscopic organisms whose combined weight amounts to about six pounds. Some of these microscopic organisms are helpful while others are harmful. These microscopic organisms serve to process our food, help with osmosis, make supplements, and protect us from us from poisons. Without them, our wellbeing is exposed to extraordinary danger. These microbes are separated from the other parts of your body by the gut lining. The lining's principle occupation is to let in important supplements from your food and keep out all the other harmful substances, for example, poisons and undigested food particles from the rest of the body.

To have a sound gut, you have to have:

Sound gut greenery, which means that you have loads of good microorganisms (probiotics) and moderately less dangerous microbes. Tight gut intersections permit only the vital nutrients to go through the gut divider obstruction and prevent harmful substances from passing through.

Without both, your system will be compromised, which would ultimately result in gut problems (and other health problems too).

Basic Gut Issues

Lamentably, for many of us, our gut wellbeing has been severely constrained by a terrible eating routine, modern fast-paced life and the abuse of prescription medicine (for e.g. anti-microbial, acid neutralizers, contraceptive pills, NSAIDs, steroids, etc), this brings about an abundance of harmful microscopic organisms and intestinal porousness, a condition called *flawed gut*. Here are probably the most widely recognized gut issues:

1. Low stomach acid

Likely causes include increased mental anxiety, which lowers acid generation from the stomach and the abuse of indigestion medications that inhibit the secretion of stomach acid. Under ideal operation, when your body can produce enough acid e.g. hydrochloric acid, the stomach's environment is mainly acidic within a certain limit of ideal conditions of proper nourishment. When the pH is as low 1, the acid destroys the greater part of the destructive microscopic organisms in food. But if you do not sufficiently generate acid, the pH can go up to 4 or 5, which may permit harmful microscopic organisms to survive and flourish inside your intestinal tract.

2. Unusual gut greenery with an excess of harmful microscopic organisms

In a solid gut, harmful organisms are constrained and firmly controlled by beneficial micro organisms. Moreover, when this beneficial foliage is destroyed and harmed, the sources relinquish their control. The usual original foliage is the yeast growth called Candida albicans. Candida disease is an immediate consequence of strange gut verdure. Basic reasons for this are; 1) over utilization of anti-infection agents (additionally found in industrially produced meats, drain, and eggs) that have a profound impact on vital microscopic organisms; and 2) an eating routine comprising foods with high sugar content, processed starches and foods that are not well matured (Matured food are rich live societies that can assist immunize the gut with great microorganisms).

A few individuals with strange gut verdure may be asymptomatic, yet some may have gastrointestinal manifestations, for example, bloating, burping, stomach agony, loose bowels and blockage.

3. Defective gut

The vast majority who have an abundance of gut verdure have some level of intestinal penetrability. The harmful microscopic organisms always release dangerous substances, which are by-products of their digestion systems. Such microbes harm the effectiveness of the gut divider hindrance, making it porous and enabling poisons to spill through. Once the poisons get assimilated into the lymph and circulation system, they cause problems in different organs in the body, particularly the brain and skin. Flawed gut has been connected with numerous brain issues like ADHD/ADD, extreme introversion, impaired learning ability, Alzheimer's, melancholy, and nervousness. Other effects are skin conditions, for example, skin break out, dermatitis, and psoriasis.

When you have a defective gut, under processed foods additionally traverse the gut divider into the circulatory system, where the body's protective system regards them as foreign and assaults them. This is the means by which sensitivity to food and intolerance arises. By and large, when the gut divider is recuperated, food hypersensitivities actually vanish. Given what we know, it is not surprising that various studies demonstrate that the deterioration of the gut plays an important role in the development of numerous immune system sicknesses like Hashimoto's, sort-1 diabetes, and rheumatoid joint inflammation. Ultimately, a cracked gut may lead to health problems as it meddles with the correct ingestion of proteins, fats, starches, B vitamins, and different micronutrients.

Regular Strategies for Healthy Gut

The human body has a fantastic capacity to mend itself, given the right assistance. Notwithstanding, patience is required as recuperation may take up to a year or two if the harm to the gut is serious. To have great general wellbeing, you initially need to mend the digestive tract, so that it can stop acting as a source of poisonous substances in the body. Secondly, you have to uproot the poisons that have now become part of your body. The following points talk on an eating regimen and way of life proposals: Consider a sans gluten diet.

It is particularly important if you have celiac infection or are gluten narrow-minded. Reduce or avoid highly processed sugar and starches in your eating routine. Stop all soft drinks, natural product juices, and caffeinated beverages. Keep away from dull vegetables and beans. These nourishments bring about a surge of insulin and an insulin-like development variable called IGF-1. IGF-1 prompts an overabundance of male hormones that cause your pores to discharge sebum, an oily substance that draws in microbes that cause skin inflammation.

Keep away from dairy. The vast majority of people with gut issues cannot process lactose (a milk sugar). Avoid dairies for 30 days and check whether your condition shows improvement. When you re-introduce dairy, begin with matured milk items, for example, yogurt, kefir, and normal crude cheeses that are generally free of lactose. This is based on the fact that that during maturation, the aging microscopic organisms devour lactose as their nourishment. Further, a small portion of individuals with a cracked gut cannot process casein (a milk protein) well. Assuming this is the case, stay away from all dairies aside from illuminated margarine or ghee, which has insignificant levels of casein or lactose. Avoid soy items unless it has been aged and is natural. Restore the correct parity of gut microscopic organisms. Eat refined dairy (yogurt, sharp cream, creme fraiche) and lacto-matured vegetables routinely. Beverage aged drinks, for example, kefir and kombucha; verify they are not sweetened with sugar. On the other hand, take an everyday probiotic supplement particularly after a course of anti-infection agents.

Purchase naturally produced meats and natural produce. Try not to keep adding to your body's lethal load by ingesting more chemicals. Drinking crisply squeezed vegetable juice will help to accelerate the body's detoxification process. For certain body sorts, it might be more fitting to have the vegetable juice with a full meal. Drink a lot of clean, filtered water -many individuals are chronically dehydrated. Hydration assists with your defecation and detoxifications. Drink large portions of water that corresponds to your weight (in pounds) in ounces. For instance, if you weigh 50 pounds, you ought to drink around 75 ounces or marginally more than nine 8-oz glasses of fluid every day. Do this consistently. The more you sweat, the more you flush the undesirable contaminants and poisons out of your pores. Additionally, consider utilizing sauna treatment for detoxification. Get a decent night's rest. This is the time your body gets the opportunity to recover and revive itself. Try to avoid stress, be upbeat. Self assured people have a tendency to have lower anxiety levels than cynics. Remind yourself to concentrate on positives thoughts. Discover ways to alleviate your anxiety. Have a go at breathing activities, meditation, jujitsu, or yoga.

CHAPTER TWO:
HOW WELL DO YOU KNOW YOUR STOMACH?

The stomach muscles are the most important parts of your body in terms of having a fine stance and complete interior wellbeing. Once your exercises and activities reduce, especially after you finish business, you hardly ever feel like reducing the amount of food you eat. This is the place stomach practices for men can be beneficial. The finest stomach activities can be done wherever you feel good and have time to perform them.

The Bicycle work out

The bicycle work out has been lately shown to be a very beneficial stomach activity. To perform it, lie on a plane surface ensuring that your lower back is pushed on the floor. Place both of your hands behind your ears and move your knees at a 45-degree position. Begin performing bicycle movements with your feet, starting slowly at first and then increasing the pace.

The Vacuum

The vacuum is fine stomach work out. It is a type of breathing activity that will manifests the best results on the more intense stomach muscles. The steps are exceptionally basic: While slowly inhaling, gradually bring your stomach segment towards your spine. Hold your body in this position for 15 seconds. Breathe out. Repeat 10 to12 times.

The Plank

The plank is an exceptional stomach exercise for men. Since this method takes concentrates on the focal piece of your body, it gives you improved quality. Lie with your face down. With your elbows, push up your body and remain in that position supported by your elbows. Hold for 40-60 seconds. Repeat 3 to 4 times.

Vertical Leg Crunch

It is a deviation of the normal crunch. This activity is very simple. Lie on your posterior on a plane surface. Put your both hands behind ears. Lift your both legs into the air, lock both legs at the feet and gradually twist your knees. Then raise your shoulders, head and upper back zone to a 30 degree position with the assistance of your abs. Backtrack gradually and repeat the same.

Chief's Chair

This is another really extraordinary sample of stomach workout is the Captain's Chair. Using a stage, grapple your feet over the casing. Holding both hands behind posterior, use your abs to drag yourself into a sitting stance. Perform this movement one or two times per week.

Rebel Dumbbell Rows

This is a really decent work out that will really work your stomach. What you really do is envision a typical push-up stance with your both hands on 2 dumbbells. You push one dumbbell upwards, and utilizing other arm to stabilize your position. Return the dumbbell to its ordinary position and repeat the step with the other arm. It is the toning down that makes this a standout amongst the most incredible stomach practices for men.

Mountain Climbers

Mountain climbers are simple to execute but are exceptionally productive work outs that essentially focus on a few regions including your abs and center area. Start in a push-up position, bring your knees up underneath midsection, and back once more. Continue with these movements until you realize the full benefits for selected areas of your stomach.

Reverse crunches

This activity will really get your stomach area buckling down. To begin this work out rest on a flat surface that is slightly raised. Perform an opposite (reverse) crunch utilizing stomach area muscles. Hold this stance for about 6 to 7 seconds before release.

Front hunches with Barbell

When many individuals mainly finish squats, they place the barbell flat on their shoulders. For this work out you will need to place the barbell in front of your head. Cross your arms and hold the barbell besides the front of your shoulder. By performing this activity, you will be using your center area to relieve you from the hunch, by focusing on your abs muscles.

Russian Twist

Russian turn is a good exercise for fortifying your stomach muscles. Begin by rests on a flat surface with knees twisted and feet level on the surface. Hold a weight and hold it in front side of the midsection while you twist back subsequently your midsection is at a 45-degree position. Twist your midsection to one side rapidly and then to the other side and then back to the initial position.

These are some best midriff practices for men that shall have a decent impact on your stomach. These stomach practices for men will offer you definition and quality. However, you must maintain a solid eating regimen and cardio routine if you want to see clearly defined six packs that you so desire.

There are a few ladies who feel that they were born trying to reduce the lump on their stomachs. They have been attempting to loose their stomach fat for so long that they rarely recall when they started doing so. The most difficult fat to dispose off is stomach fat. This stomach fat appears to mock its owner - seemingly suggesting that whatever one does, it cannot gotten rid of. It is difficult to find a lady who has not at one time or another sought information on how to loose stomach fat.

It is every ladies dream to be able to have a flat tummy so that they would wear tight fitting blouses or t-shirts. Unfortunately, nature has it so that it is easier for ladies to accumulate fat in their tummies, which when accumulated, may be hard to remove.

Many ladies have read many books that talk about reduction of fat and have tried many of the techniques explained therein. Some have gone to extraordinary lengths to achieve this but have ended up causing more harm that good to their bodies.

There are many unsafe chemicals and manufactured medications that claim to do wonders and almost miraculously help in removing stomach fat through the use of strange formulations or concoctions. Many of these may end up causing bodily and even mental harm in the long run.

Many ladies have ended spending tons of cash in a bid to bid farewell to stomach fat, not to mention the time and effort spent in doing so. However, many ladies have ended up loosing the fight against stomach fat. Ladies don't like thrashing and thus they try it with retribution. They have made a promise, specifically, to not let stomach fat ruin their possibility of living a better life. Ladies will do anything to get rid of stomach fat.

The most noticeably thing about stomach fat is that it looks revolting and may negatively affect a person's wellbeing. There is a known connection between dangers to wellbeing, for instance, cardio-vascular sicknesses, heart infirmities, diabetes and hyper-pressure in individuals who have relatively more fat on their stomach. While at present you may not be overly concerned about the way you look, you may still end up being haunted and disturbed by issues concerning your wellbeing. This concern may be the drive that drives you to want to loose stomach fat.

If you have been pondering on what is the genuine mystery on the best way to condition your stomach and get truly tight abs, then this is the chapter for you. I will let you know why you are not getting a flat stomach and perhaps what you are doing incorrectly. I am writing this for those who are serious on getting a flat stomach and to find out what you ought to be doing, instead of what you may wrongly spending your time on doing wondering why you are getting nowhere.

One of the first things you ought to know about conditioning your stomach is that abs exercises alone will never get you flat abs. The issue is that many people have been told time and again that doing stomach muscle activities will get them six-pack abs. This is so distant from reality. I've said it in past articles and I will say it once more: abdominal muscle activities do not produce enough energy to burn fat in order to produce six-pack abs. The best way to burn fat is to figure out how to do full body workouts to amplify your metabolic surge. This is the fundamental reason that abdominal muscle workouts will never get you past a certain point. They will fortify your abs, yet never dispose of the fat over them.

Further, another common error is where everybody advised to do heaps of cardio workouts. We are informed that the more you do your cardio schedules the more calories you burn. Ugh! Think about all the time you are squandering doing long, exhausting cardio workouts when you could be doing activities that are a great deal more efficient in burning fat. Truth be told, if you happen to do interim preparation schedules, then you will see vastly improved and snappier results than doing cardio. Interim preparation includes both high-force workouts, consolidated with low-power workouts done on an interim premise.

Another huge error made by many people regarding the reduction of stomach fat and which is at times attributed to supernatural causes is the utilization of pills. There are currently many advertisements that publicize the use of synthetic pills. Those who know me are aware of the fact that I loathe prepared synthetic pill. I have never understood why some people decide to spend such a great amount of cash on eating routine pills, when they could spend considerably less on activities and schedules that are more beneficial for their lives. This book shall enable you to make much healthier decisions in this regard.

Finally, here is one final tip regarding the most proficient method to condition your stomach - abandoning the abdominal muscle machines. There are several contraptions available today for removing stomach fat but I need to let you know that none of them will get you a flat stomach. While some may help you reach a certain point, they will never enable you to sufficiently burn the fat from your midsection. Here, I give my apologies; I know loads of individuals who have purchased these devices. The funny thing is that most of them wind up in carport deals. If in any case you do not believe me, glance around and you will find this to be true!

CHAPTER THREE:
YOUR SECOND BRAIN AND THE CHEMISTRY OF ADDICTION

At the point when your striving to get more fit and you see that your arms and legs are getting more slender and even your face is looking more appealing, it can be baffling when you observe that your stomach fat is not reducing.

Enthusiastic Weight Gain/Weight Loss - Believe it or not, your feelings are an indispensable piece of your weight reduction process - notwithstanding for the unshakable paunch fat that just does not seem to go away. When it continues sticking around, your feelings can begin to negatively affect your framework. You feel low, disappointed, and then...you fall into bad eating habits due to frustrations. Control those feelings – be positive and focus on your objectives. Concentrate on your prosperity - not your disappointments.

Wash Away Your Waist Line – in order to begin the process of burning your stomach fat, you have to begin your day with 6 to 8 glasses of water. I know - it sounds insane, yet one of the reasons that the stomach fat is staying around is a result of poisons in your body. Water washes out the poisons and gives your body a simple and common solution for flushing your system.

This will cause your stomach to be filled and purify your body. Further, your body will lessen its tendency to clutch at fatty substances. Avoid sweet sugary beverages. If you cannot drink plain water, then you can add some bit of sugar squash into the water for added flavor.

Vitamins are vital (see the word essential in vitamin...think that is a mishap?) When you go on an eating regimen of any kind - or begin upsetting your body science, you have to ensure that your body is getting the nutrients that are important to for optimum function.. You can begin with a decent multi-vitamin, and may need to add some extra vitamins in view of what you are battling with. Vitamin B gives you that much needed jolt of energy. Vitamin C is essential for battling off diseases and colds. Garlic is a characteristic anti-toxin and can help keep your body fit as a fiddle.

No Exercise Weight Loss? (Truly - would you truly like to attempt that?) The thought of doing nothing and getting everything sounds great but this is a major joke. It simply doesn't work that way. Your body needs to burn calories. You increase the rate of burning calories by doing stuff. Walk, run, hop, skip, or undertake routine activities such as cleaning the house etc., whatever it is - simply get moving.

Focus on 10-15 minutes of activity a day until you feel the need to increase the time spent for activities. Do not avoid or postpone the process of relieving yourself. Doing so can bring about problems of blockages.

Do not overstuff your stomach. The normal healthy stomach is the size of a normal man's crunched hand. Focus on healthy parts, extending the internal stomach size can bring about long term effects. You will burn your stomach fat in a very short duration.

Jolt Your Diet

Since inspiration is so pivotal to keeping to an eating regimen, I suggest that you think of some eating regimen help that will help you get past the most difficult part - the starting!

The way to getting in shape in the long term is to take new initiatives for physical action and adopting better eating regimens. You can get more fit by picking the right nourishments and the right activities. However - the starting is hard and the need to have some early achievement is critical to keeping up the pace. To truly kick off your goals and get your inspiration pumping, you can attempt what I did, which helped shed the pounds. Apart from helping you to initially lose 15 lbs rapidly, it supports your vitality by wiping out the poisons that are in your colon. The best part – this can be done at virtually no cost.

A large number of people experience the bad effects of many stomach related issues and depend on medications that not only have adverse reactions or effects but also cost a fortune. There are approaches to manage these illnesses without utilizing medications. A large portion of these issues stem from an eating routine, which affects our wellbeing drives us to take anti-toxins or acid neutralizers to "settle" the issue.

Do we realize that when our body needs too much acidic food or drinks in it our entire framework is traded off? An acidic environment initiates the breakdown of vulnerable systems which can then prompt a variety of issues. Aside from issues that are already identified, if the pH of your blood is below 7.3, then your body seeks a basic substance to bring about a balance.

If in any chance you are not supporting your body with basic nourishments and refreshments, then your body will search out whatever it can cure increased acidity. Where do you think our body stores significant antacid material? Your bones and teeth are basically a calcium bank. If you recollect your high school chemistry, you shall recall that calcium is soluble. Our bodies are unbelievably ingenious and will do whatever they have to in order to restore pH balance. The calcium in our bones and teeth are ransacked to keep our blood pH in balance.

Disposing of stomach fat and acquiring stomach abs is a fantasy for the vast majority. One could take after an amazing workout regimen and eating routine arrangement and get perfect abs quickly. There are numerous books and eating routine arranges that can help you do this. However, many people who seek after ripped abs fail to see the underlying causes of stomach fat.

The reason the vast majority is overweight and has high muscle to fat ratio ratios is first due to their diets which comprise of highly processed fatty or oily foods. Secondly, they live sedentary lives with few engaging activities. These are the main drivers of the vast majority's stomach fat.

The above reasons should be the first areas to be tackled if one is to shed some pounds. The reason that many people do not is because it takes longer than other methods. However, if pursued for a long time, a slender body can be maintained with little or no activity.

Clearly the first thing that needs to change is the decisions you make. It's as straightforward as picking squeeze over pop and plain popcorn over treat. For instance, you have to take the initiative of eating more veggies and reduced protein levels. You don't need to do sample things all the time yet major exercise is invested in major change in body science can be achieved more than once.

Next you have to get somewhat more active. Do things as basic as taking the stairs rather than the lift once per week, as well as stopping in the back of the parking area so hopefully you need to walk more distant (wellbeing allowing), or even simply going for a walk a few times every week.

Next, you have to become more active. There are a few basic but engaging activities you can do. For instance, climbing the stairs instead of climbing the lift at least once per week, parking your car further so that you can walk a longer distance, or going for a walk a few times each week.

Such apparently basic activities can have beneficial outcomes in the long term since you shall loose fat and improve your overall wellbeing. The change begins with you changing your disposition on life.

The most direct response to these inquiries is basic. Consuming soluble water does not hurt your stomach nor does your stomach wipe out the advantages of antacid (regularly likewise alluded to as ionized water).

Let's take a couple of minutes to comprehend why this bodes well for us. In the first place we should discuss how the stomach functions. Within our stomachs can be an acidic domain that has a practically unending supply of extra acid assets which are accessible when required straightaway by means of the stomach divider. The acid is utilized to eliminate microorganisms and infections that accompany food intakes. As indicated by Sang Wang, the creator of "Converse Aging", "The stomach pH worth kept up at around 4. When we eat food and beverage water, particularly antacid water, the pH esteem inside the stomach goes up. At the point when this happens, there is an input instrument in our stomach to recognize this and summons the stomach divider to discharge more hydrochloric acid into the stomach to take the pH esteem back to 4." So, with this criticism component instantly killing, drinking ionized water appears like an acts of futility, isn't that so? In no way, shape or form!

The solution for our situation comes in the way the stomach divider makes hydrochloric acid. As indicated by prominent confusion, our stomach is always acidic. This is not always the case. If there was a chance that there was a pocket of acid anyplace in our body in the long run it would burn a gap through the range. Along these lines, as Sang Wang clarifies, "The cells in our stomach divider must deliver hydrochloric acid on a right away, as-required premise."

The components that are utilized by the stomach cell to make hydrochloric acid are carbon dioxide, water, and sodium chloride.

And every single mixture, as we learn in elementary science as kids, must be changed regularly. Along these lines, when the stomach produces hydrochloric acid, "The by-product of making hydrochloric acid is sodium bicarbonate or potassium bicarbonate. The HCl is discharged into the stomach and the by-item is discharged into the circulatory system".

These bicarbonates are the antacid cushions that neutralize excess acids in the blood; they break up strong acid waste into a fluid form. As they neutralize this excess acidity, the excess sodium bicarbonate and potassium bicarbonate are converted into carbon dioxide which is transported to the lungs and afterward released. When we eat food, our stomach divider produces acid, and then it sends basic substances through our blood to kill acid outside of our stomach. In the meantime, carbon dioxide gas is discharged from our lungs.

Consequently, the start considered solving of the soluble water as precise, however as we look more carefully, our inexplicable bodies respond consummately so that when we drink ionized water, the alkalinity is passed easily into our circulation system, alongside those antacid parts. As Sang Wang clarifies, "Soluble or acid delivered by the body must have an equivalent and inverse acid or basic created by the body; in this manner, keeping the laws of science in equalization. Be that as it may, basic supplied from outside the body, such as drinking antacid water, brings about a net increase of alkalinity in our body."

You can, hence, drink soluble water at any time of the day. In case you drink the water when your stomach is full, the alkalinity is goes into your circulatory system with the basic supports. When you drink with a void stomach, the water finds nothing to interact with and passes into the circulatory system.

CHAPTER FOUR:
THE FOODS TO EAT FOR A HEALTHY GUT

It is basic knowledge that you can strip that midsection fat by doing the right exercises. But do you know that you can eat your way to a flat stomach? I know it sounds amazing, however it is conceivable to lose tummy swell and obtain washboard abs by devouring fat! The wellbeing and wellness specialists at Prevention magazine absolutely appear to agree with this. If you eat certain sorts of food, you should have the capacity to consume with burning heat those tummy calories genuine quick without needing to take plan of action to crunches and stomach turns.

Some of the things you can eat for a flat stomach include olives, avocado, nuts and seeds. To focus on the fat around your stomach, you need to eat food rich in MUFA or monounsaturated fatty acids – this is an exceptionally useful fat. You need to hand pick and select from the 5 fundamental gatherings of MUFA and incorporate them in your meals.

A significant amount of MUFA can be found in oils like soybean oil, walnut oil, pea nut oil, sesame oil, flax seed oil, safflower oil, olive oil, canola oil, rice wheat oil and also in pesto sauce. These are the oils with which you ought to cook your food. Avoid sunflower oil. Olives are especially good if you want your swelling tummy or pot paunch vanish. Take your pick from green olive tapenade, dark olive tapenade, new green or dark olives.

Building up a regimen comprising of the right nourishment to eat to reduce heartburn and continuing with the regimen is the first step towards recuperating from indigestion sickness. It can be difficult to distinguish the right food to eat for indigestion and then continuing with it.

In the first place, you may not know the right food to eat for indigestion, particularly if you do not know which nourishments are causing your heartburn and related effects. In fact, indigestion may not even be the cause of these effects. You could be encountering an undesirable reaction to a given food as opposed to indigestion.

Importantly, diagnosing your eating routine remains your best alternative for distinguishing a dietary arrangement. Through experimentation, you ought to have the capacity to distinguish what nourishment to eat to avoid the effects of heartburn.

The main thing you have to do is to find which nourishments are causing these undesirable effects. Similarly as with any eating routine, you ought to start by avoiding nourishments that are an issue for you. While it can indeed be hard to adore some of those foods you adore so much, you need to figure out how to identify alternative foods that offer provide reduce indigestion but still provide solid nourishments your body.

Liven up your eating routine by fusing new flavors into your food while at the same time checking off the foods that cause your particular digestive problems. You will most likely find foods that are prone to cause heartburn in your digestive system.

A complete and comprehensive list of the nourishments that each indigestion sufferer ought to stay away from essentially does not exist. You need to know that a food rundown is customized to your condition. You will need to consolidate foods that you have dependably eaten into your new solid and adjusted eating routine.

Luckily, there are usually accessible nourishments that for the most part are connected with heartburn alleviation for many people. These foods do not bring about indigestion and alternate manifestations of heartburn. Foods that are low in acid have a tendency to assuage heartburn side effects. Organic products with low acid levels, for example, apples and bananas ought to be a piece of your eating routine. Most heartburn sufferers endure vegetables, for example, broccoli, carrots, cabbage, green beans and peas. The vast majority of heartburn sufferers can safely eat a solid mixture of grains and meat. These foods help in neutralizing stomach acidity.

What to eat for a flat stomach. Note that these are foods that you ought to eat regardless of the possibility that you have a flat stomach. Try not to stop eating these sound nourishments when you dispose off the stiff-necked gut fat. If in case quit eating these foods, there is a high chance that you will get the fat right back on your tummy. Try not to do it.

Normal nuts like almonds. Eat lots of nuts such as almonds. However, do not eat them salted. Get used to consuming them in their natural state.. Nuts are a great source of protein. Furthermore, they ordinarily contain cell reinforcements such as Vitamin E which help battle bad chemicals in your body. This helps you get a flat stomach.

Sound oils. Utilizing oils like natural virgin olive oil and natural coconut oil can help you lose stomach fat. Avoid hydrogenated or incompletely hydrogenated oils that are found in numerous nourishments nowadays. Hydrogenated oils are bad for your entire body. Stay far from them in your quest to get a flat stomach.

Common Peanut spread. You must utilize regular nutty spread in light of the fact that it contains healthier oils than non-characteristic nutty spread. You do not need hydrogenated oils in your nutty spread. Check the ingredients to verify this fact. Nutty spread is an incredible source of protein and vitamins. It will help keep you full. You can also consume it with specific vegetables such as Celery and Bok Choy.

Avocados. Although Avocados contain fat, it's solid fat. It's filling and it has bunches of fiber. Avocados put solid filling in your tummy and make it simpler to stay away from bad nourishment.

Cruciferous vegetables. Eat veggies like Bok Choy, Brussels sprouts, and Broccoli. They are high in cancer prevention agents and will help you get a flat stomach due to cell reinforcements which battle pesticides and chemicals in your body.

4 foods to look for to keep your stomach lean, soothed—and even cancer-free

There are certainly some foods which you should avoid completely or do so sparingly. These include cakes, treats, sugary beverages (including business commercial organic juices), most processed breakfast grains, and most white foodstuffs, for example, bread, sugar and rice. Foods which should be avoided include pan-fried fast foods and foods cooked in commercial cooking oil (Trans fats).

The white flour and sugary items separate are rapidly absorbed in your body and increase your glucose levels. Consequently, your body produces insulin to adjust your sugar. Insulin is a stockpiling hormone, which stores fat for crises. One of the spots it stores the fat is on your stomach.

If this continues frequently and for a long time, your body experiences difficulty in creating the insulin needed to control your glucose. This is the point where your pancreas fails and may lead to diabetes. So continually eating the wrong food can deliver these two genuine symptoms alongside various other health issues. The net result is that you become bigger and unhealthier - not what you are hoping to do.

The take-away foods and snacks are always cooked in trans fats, found in most manufactured cooking oil, which load up your body with manufactured man-made fats that have no medical advantages. They increase your cholesterol and load up your body with fat that settles around your liver and your stomach, among other places. There is a fair chance that such foods have been adding to your stomach fat over the years.

Nourishments to Eat

There are foods that contribute to having a flat stomach. These are foods include incline meat, fish, beans, nuts, leafy foods. The formulas you can apply to cake various combinations of these foods is only constrained by your creative imagination. Indeed, there is likely more data about various cooking formulas and combinations than there has ever been. Numerous cooks and nourishment pros are investigating on solid eating methodologies and utilizing regular combinations.

In any case, for these foods to work, you do need to work out improvements in the manner you prepare these foods. With good food combinations, you will be shocked how rapidly you begin to lose your stomach fat. You should concentrate on how you are going to roll out the improvements. While there may be initial drawbacks, yet this is a small price to pay in light of the benefits you stand to gain of stomach fat diminish and improving your wellbeing.

You can make a move now by supplanting the fat creating foods you have been eating for a long time with solid, flat stomach nourishments and appreciate looking and feeling better through your 50s and past.

You can get the attractive stomach you have been envisioning about without even a crunch. Most likely you are asking yourself "how could this happen? Perhaps I must do crunches in order to realize my goal of attaining a flat stomach."Wrong! There are 5 focal methodologies that will make your stomach reduce and become flat.

1-STOP being fixated on crunches

Your abs are not made to flex which is the main thing that happens amid crunches - so fundamentally they are pointless. Your abs are made to settle or balance your whole body while strolling, running, and taking a seat, etc. Therefore, they ought to be prepared to undertake these activities. Notwithstanding amid doing thrusts (which are extraordinary lower body works out) your abs attempt to balance out you. For instance, incase you put your hands over your head while doing jumps, you will realize that you could make a significantly better lurch. What does this let you know? It lets you know that amid all these various activities whether normal activities or induced exercises such as push ups, crunches and other, your abs serve to ensure that your body is balanced . Hence, undertaking normal activities can develop your abs even when not doing induced exercises such as crunches.

2 - Work on the guideline of muscle over-burden

What do I mean by that? I imply that in case you are lifting weights or doing body weight activities and you have a feeling that can do 25-35 raps without a much of a struggle, then your muscles are not getting sufficient challenge. At this stage you ought to add some more weight. If say, you are used to hold 5 pound (2.2 kg) dumbbells each time you are doing presses and you can do 20 or 30 raps effortlessly, then you would never have the capacity to build your muscles. What you have to do is to gradually add weights to your schedule. For instance, if you are doing pushups and they get to simple, then you need to ensure that you make it harder on yourself. One strategy for making it harder while doing pushups is to put your feet on a seat; this would make the pushups more difficult. Never let your normal routine get too simple, if this happens, then you need to make it harder to accomplish the same routine.

3-Cardio preparing should be difficult too

Interim preparation is one approach to do your cardio all the more difficult. I you have seen individuals in the rec center strolling on the treadmill with 3 miles for every hour or thereabouts while also watching a show on the TV. This is a good example of what should not be doing if you are to realize positive changes. You have to do interim preparation where you shift the test of your cardiovascular schedule. For instance, to expand your heartbeat by running very fast for 2 minutes, strolling for a short while and repeating the fast run again.

4-Your Diet

That is truly where the abs are made. You MUST watch your eating routine; you MUST watch what you eat. I am not a major fan of tallying calories although I tried it out in the past without much success. My tip to you is to check fixings. Take a look at the ingredients written in the container. It is by far better to consume foods that do not have ingredients written on them, for instance, leafy foods - this means that you are consuming solid food for which you do not have to stress over any calories or fats. In case you consume food you are in a situation of inconvenience (e.g. when traveling), try to eat food with as little harmful (or unknown) ingredients as possible.

5-Get a bolster group

My fifth tip to you is to get a bolster group. In case you feel like it is difficult to do this as an individual think about joining kind of a group such as a forum, a class, a blog, a discussion on the web, or essentially find a workout partner. The most important point is to find a constructive person with similar interests or hobbies. Trust me, you can go far if you have such a partner who supports you and cheers you up each time you feel low or feel like surrendering.

There are very many diet methodologies that advance great hopes for weight reduction. Do you realize that basically eating fat burning diets could be pretty much as successful as an eating routine?

The body has a unique response to any meal - be it small nibble or larger quantities. Dietary specialists have acquired the capacity to analyze certain body responses to a variety of healthy foods that really help calorie counters to burn off excess calories and become more fit. With no insane standards, rules, or eating regimen regulations, calorie counters can enjoy a variety of fat burning food choices keeping in mind that the end goal is to obtain better weight reduction results more quickly.

What Qualifies as Fat Burning Foods

As dietary specialists constantly endeavor to distinguish the primary nourishments that help health food partakers to get more fit, current reports state that the most effective fat burning food things can be found in gatherings, for example,

High protein, low sugar foods, particularly inclines meats, fish, beans, and nuts.

High fiber foods, particularly entire grain servings, for example, cocoa rice, fiber oat with no added substances and sugars, organic products, and vegetables.

Foods rich in water, particularly leafy foods.

Why Certain Foods Help Burn Fat

In looking at the various weight reduction advantages of every classification, dietitians state that the body's interesting digestive procedures and responses to these fat burning foods are the key focus points in helping health food fans to dispose off muscle to fat quotients.

Eating Lean, High Protein Foods

Premier, high protein nourishments that are low in sugars have been demonstrated to help burn fat. This is because protein-rich foods help the consumers to have a feeling of a full stomach. As the body gradually processes proteins, the body really holds at other nutrients for a longer period.

When the body stays full, health food recipients have the capacity to control hunger, food

47

cravings, and enticements better. By diminishing and controlling one's general admission of nourishment, the body will eventually start to seek other options in order to maintain vitality. To fuel natural needs, the body is compelled to go through fat stockpiling ranges for "fuel," bringing about weight reduction. Therefore, a solid admission and controlled serving of incline proteins with every meal and for the duration of the day can help weight watchers to experience upgraded fat burning advantages!

Expending High Fiber, Fat Burning Foods

Notwithstanding protein rich nourishments, high fiber foods, particularly naturally grown products furnish the body with a more beneficial capacity to burn off fat. Like protein, fiber travels through the digestive tract gradually, bringing about greater feelings of fullness. Notably, fiber really expands the stomach and digestive tract once it blends with the body's digestive juices. When the fiber foods expand, the stomach actually feels more full - regardless of the fact that a person may have consumed just a relatively smaller serving of food.. Accordingly, weight watchers can control their levels of appetite and food consumed and eventually utilize the energy of fat cells to give their bodies vital jolts of energy.

Liquids as Fat Burning Foods?

Additionally, when endeavoring to burn off muscle to fat ratios, one of the most basic methods of expending calories is to assimilate more liquids and water into one's eating routine. By avoiding sugar-upgraded refreshments, for example, soft drinks, fake juices, and mixed beverages, the body has the capacity keep up the burning of solid fat.

If you are attempting to get more fit and tone up, you may have noticed that the most troublesome part of your body to tone up is your stomach. The muscles on your lower stomach area are basically like jam. If you cannot stand this anymore, you need to make a move.

You could take the option of having a tummy tuck. However, many people cannot afford this due to cost implications. For some people this may be the main option of having a flat stomach. Reasons for having loose skin among some ladies may occur after giving birth or perhaps after loosing a lot of weight. If you fall under this category, you may need to counsel your family doctor. He or she refer you to a plastic surgeon..

You can get a flat stomach by sticking to your special regimen steadfastly for the initial first two weeks from starting. If you have arrangements to meet family and companions for a feast, you may have to reschedule the event if you feel that it shall compromise your regimen. You can reschedule to meet for a feast at a later date.

You should sit down and work out the objectives you plan to accomplish. Your number one objective is getting a flat stomach. You should work out and stick to it. You should eat sound food and stick to it. You should keep a diary of the foods you eat. Along these lines, you can note down the days or weeks when you shed pounds and when you put on weight. When you recognize what foods and nourishment mixes are making you put on weight, you can remove them of your eating routine or seek alternatives.

With a specific end goal being that of getting a flat stomach you should dispose of all the junk food in your home. When you develop cravings, the temptation to eat junk food may overwhelm the desire to have a flat stomach. If you fall for this temptation, you might end up feeling guilty. You can eliminate this cycle completely by eliminating junk food from your house or by giving it away. Verify you dispose of any commercial foodstuffs too. This include TV suppers, artificial squeezed meats, pre-made dinners, and so on. Just eat fresh solid home cooked meals made with crisp fixings.

Fill your kitchen with naturally grown products. However, take care that these are always fresh otherwise they may have effects that are worse than junk food. Simply go to the market and replenish finished stock. You need to add healthy foods to your eating regimen comprising of multigrain, wholegrain nourishments and incline proteins.

Ensure that you exercise for not less than one hour daily. You will need to do cardio workouts that incorporate strolling, running, swimming, etc. You will need to add weight lifting to your normal exercises too. Crunches, leg lifts and sit-ups are magnificent ways to help you tone up your stomach and finally acquire that flat stomach that you are working at.

The 8 best foods for your gut: Your immune system will sing when you work these

Developing studies show that a good biological environment is made up of billions of useful microorganisms living in your body, which form a key part of a person's general wellbeing. This can lessen the danger of a variety of illnesses - including irritation, joint inflammation, coronary illness, tumor, and even dementia - and help improve muscle to fat quotients and thus maintaining solid weight.

However, to keep up this sensitive biological community of useful microorganisms, the majority of which lives in your gut, you have to nourish them regularly. Anything with probiotics, that is, beneficial microbes, can help improve the essence of wellbeing. Here are the food items that can accomplish this:

Yogurt

The lord of probiotics, this dairy item is the best bet for gainful microorganisms. Whether you like Greek or normal, low-fat or full-fat, what matters is the presence of "live dynamic societies", which means the availability of good microbes. While you can take plain natural yoghurt or incorporate several mixes in your yoghurt, be sure not to exceed 15 grams of sugar for every serving - any more than that, and you will simply be giving the more harmful gut microorganisms with the sugar they cherish.

Kefir

Like yogurt, this aged milk beverage is smooth, slightly tart, and rich in many probiotics. Additionally, lactose is minimal (one percent or less) which makes it perfect for individuals who are allergic to lactose (start with a little amount just to test your reaction). In addition, kefir comprises anywhere in the range of 8 to 11 grams of protein for each container and only 100 calories. Thus, it serves to give you a feeling of fullness, which is good during a diet regimen.

Miso Paste

Dairy products are not the only sources probiotics. Miso paste is produced using matured and aged soybeans and is crammed with great microscopic organisms. Accessible in an assortment of hues and flavors, this low-calorie foodstuff is an excellent method of including a natural, appetizing flavor to your meals. It is likewise loaded with protein, fiber, and vitamin K. Miso is perfect for coating fish or chicken before cooking, blending into panfry, or adding to fluids to make a miso juices. However, it is important to note that it may have a high level of sodium.

Tempeh

Representing aged soybeans, this mixed bag is accessible in a cake-like structure, and offers a nuttier option to tofu. It can be used as part of sandwiches, mixed fries, or even marinated and flame broiled foods. Beside probiotics, tempeh contains around 15 grams of protein for each half-glass and is a decent source of iron. Like most soy items, it can help lessen cholesterol.

Kombucha Tea

Kombucha Tea is fizzy, tart, and with slight vinegar-like taste. It is increasingly becoming a popular beverage with health benefits. The tea is normally carbonated by "scoby", a particulate matter that is the main source of microbes and yeast that make up the probiotics. It is better to purchase it from the store than to make it yourself because its preparation process can be quite involving. It follows a maturation process similar to that of liquor. Therefore, it is advisable to consume not more than one 12-oz bottle day by day.

Sauerkraut

A famous sauce for franks, this matured cabbage has antiquated roots as a source of probiotics. For true probiotic muscle, avoid canned sauerkraut, the fact that it is pasteurized means that the healthy bacteria have been killed off. Instead, make your own homemade sauerkraut in a crock.

Sourdough Bread

This chewy bread gets its eminently acrid tinge from lactic acid starter, which provides a strain of microorganisms called lactobacillus, a vital probiotic. Sourdough is additionally a good choice for those with diabetes since its rich fiber and entire grain makeup help diminish glucose spikes.

Super nourishments are increasingly being viewed favorably globally due to their medical advantages and the capacity to help people to get into shape. These characteristic foods go past the "normal" assortment because they are rich in phytochemicals and cancer prevention agents. They slow down the aging process and help your body become leaner and healthier.

Here are the ten best foods for weight reduction and why they give all that you have to ideal wellbeing.

1. Blueberries

These yummy little berries are rich in cell reinforcements. Full of flavonoids and proanthocyandins, they help in strengthening memory and cognizance. A prominent expansion to any fat misfortune program, they taste incredible threw together in a low fat smoothie, utilized as a part of entire wheat hotcakes or biscuits or just to add another measurement to your natural product serving of mixed greens.

2. Broccoli

Broccoli has a wealth of wellbeing boosting properties. It contains isothiocyanantes, which activates the body's generation of tumor battling proteins. It has as much calcium as a glass of milk and more vitamin C than an orange. Also, it is one of the greatest sources of vitamin A in any organic product or vegetable. The main catch is you do need to eat it raw to realize its benefits. If you cannot eat it deal with it raw, you can gently steam it before preparation. You can serve it together with a serving of mixed greens or mixing it through entire wheat noodles.

3. Ginger

Utilized all through history for therapeutic purposes, ginger helps to ensure against disease in addition to boosting the vulnerable systems. It helps battle contamination in our body, builds digestive chemical action and is one of the characteristic weight reduction foods that accelerate the digestion system and burn fat. Ginger is also a prevalent solution for sickness and is especially good for pregnant women. You can take hot ginger tea with a shower of nectar or use in Asian mix fries and mesh a bit through solid marinades and sauces.

4. Linseeds

Linseeds contain the key omega 3 fatty acids, which decrease cholesterol. However, are they hostile to growth and can help bring menopausal symptoms? They promote wellbeing and help one remain calm. One tablespoon of linseeds a day will give you the omega 3 fats that you require. Sprinkle them over your grain or blend through soups and meals. Linseeds should be stored in a refrigerator or freezer.

5. Oats

Comprising of substantial amounts of dissolvable fiber, oats help lower cholesterol levels and enhance the health of the entrails. They have a low GI (glycaemic file) which implies that they make the ideal breakfast to supercharge your day. Oats are a prevalent suggestion in most health improvement plans.

6. Salmon

Salmon are a phenomenal source of omega 3 fats, protein and vitamin D. Solid fat projects prescribe eating salmon twice per week, as it reduces triglyceride levels. Any remaining calories that your body does not burn are transformed into triglycerides, which are a kind of fat. Poach or flame broil salmon, and present with a verdant plate of mixed greens or steamed vegetables. Combine tinned salmon with squashed sweet potatoes to make nutritious patties - kids just adore them.

7. Soy

Soy protein contains cell reinforcement isoflavones which neutralize the development of cholesterol in veins, diminishing the danger of heart assault and blood clusters. It is good for maintaining healthy bones and forestalling osteoporosis. Ensure that you select soy items that are organically grown as opposed to genetically modified ones. Use soy protein or tofu rather than burgers and chicken in formulas. Use soy drain over your grain or in natural product smoothies.

8. Tea

Various studies have demonstrated that the effective cell reinforcement polyphenols in tea diminish the danger of diseases furthermore lower cholesterol levels. What's more, drinking tea helps bring down the anxiety hormone cortisol. Green tea specifically has had much discourse with respect to its weight reduction advantages. Really all teas contain polyphenols and in this way all have positive advantages. Ideally, drink your tea without milk to get the most advantage.

9. Tomatoes

Tomatoes, which are low in calories, are a flexible wellbeing cognizant element for any health improvement plan. Simply add tomatoes to your pasta sauce to help your cell reinforcement admission and to bring down your danger of endless infections, especially prostate malignancy. They are rich in lycopene, which battles harmful free radicals and are also rich in vitamin C. There are such a variety of energizing ways to incorporate tomatoes into your meals. Whether it is pureed into sauces, cleaved through summer servings of mixed greens or tossed into an entire wheat tortilla, this marvelous foodstuff is an unquestionable requirement.

10. Yogurt

Yogurt is a favorite of many weight watchers. Not just does its rich surface help fulfill cravings, it is an extraordinary source of calcium, protein, vitamin B12 and riboflavin. In addition it contains probiotics that create a healthy gut and strengthen overall resistance to disease. Use sugar free, low fat yogurt as a substitute for cream in sauces, curries, and sweets. It is phenomenal as a 'snappy nibble' on the run and can be cooked in both flavorful and sweet formulas.

Ensure that you consolidate these ten best nourishments for weight reduction into your week-by-week weight reduction eating arrangements to realize the expanded vitality and boundless medical advantages.

What is the most important thing I tell my companions when they ask what the best foodstuffs are for a flat stomach? I tell them that that their dietary patterns do not have to comply with any of the most recent eating regimens... - "low carb" or "low fat", or high this or low that as such is not the ideal approach to significantly loose muscle to fat quotients to get extraordinary abs. The most ideal path is to streamline things a bit. Attaining overall balance is important. For instance, apart to establishing a healthy eating routine, it is more beneficial to incorporate supplements made up rich foods in their rawest form.

Usually, it is the manner in which foods are handled that causes problems in our bodies. Most nourishments in their crude state are indeed excellent. However, there are a few exemptions of course. For instance, it is important to know foods that may be harmful or even poisonous in their raw state for instance, some varieties of mushrooms.

So here are some important realities about your eating routine and foods that will help you to get fit and develop awesome abs!

1. Get a lot of good protein in your day-by-day diet. Protein will make you feel fulfilled for more. What's more, it's a building piece for keeping up and building awesome abs. Additionally, remember that the amount of muscles you have is a standout amongst the most important components for controlling your digestion system.

2. When it comes to carbs, ensure that the majority of your sugar admission is from high fiber foods, for example, veggies, organic product, and foul grains. It is best to evade refined sugars and grains. I would search for carb sources that have no less than 2-3 grams of fiber for every 10 grams of aggregate starch.

3. Many people individuals attempt to eat too little fat in their eating regimen. However, this could have a negative impact on your hormone levels. You need to ingest some solid fat daily from sources such as nuts and seeds, avocados, olive oil, and eggs.

In case you need to lose that stomach fat and have that perfectly flat tummy, the best foods for you are out there just waiting to be found. In the meantime you may be trying to loose stomach fat with the wrong type of foods, which you otherwise believe (or were made to believe) is good for you.

For example, you would not argue with anyone that soy good. But this may not be wholly true because diets comprising unfermented soy should not be consumed because they could even add to stomach fat if consumed in large amounts. Soy is simply one more nourishment food and yet it is not wellbeing food. The advertising business which promotes individuals who know diet foods have helped individuals to accept their lies about what healthy nourishments are and what foods would really save them money.

Adhering to a good diet should be exhausting. There is an unending list of solid nourishments that could help you lose your stomach fats. There are essential foods in the kitchen that could suffice for solid foods and that are good for you. One example is eggs. You may have been made to believe that entire eggs (whites and yolks) are undesirable. Others may tell you to drop the yolk and eat the remainder. However, what remains of the egg after disposing the yolk? The answer is that nothing does! More than 90% of all supplements of an egg are on the yolks, and eating the whites only is wasteful since you loose all the nutrients and money too!

While it was once unfortunately considered as fattening, the coconut has recaptured its place as a fat-burning wellbeing food. Whether it is the milk or the juice, a coconut is a food that really improves a person's wellbeing. Indeed, even coconut oil is a beneficial cooking oil. A few nuts such as almonds, pecans and walnuts are similarly solid foods that promote the burning of stomach fat.

Losing midsection fats is truly about knowing and eating the best nourishments for you. Delving into research on the procedures that can or cannot help you loose fat around the stomach is also vital. A flat stomach does not simply mean a solid body, it also bears a relationship with increased prosperity and a sound perspective on life issues.

What is your favorite food? You may need to say farewell to it for some time due to your weight reduction program. However, in the course of your weight reduction program, you are bound to discover alternative foods that shall quickly become your favorites – replacing previous favorites that were otherwise unhealthy.

The best nourishments for weight reduction are the kinds of foods that will help you to control cravings, accelerate the digestion system, ease assimilation, and expand vitality.

While considering the best foods for weight reduction, you ought to additionally consider removing foods that would promote fat cell development. Avoid eating foods with sugar, fat, and prepared packaged foods. Effects of beverages are hardly noticeable when consuming fewer calories. Water is the best drink for shedding pounds. Refreshments made from ground juices and smoothies are good alternatives to sugar filled beverages. Pop and caffeinated beverages are incredible foods for fat cells.

10 Best Foods for Weight Loss

1 .Sprouts, grown beans, vegetables, and seeds, are   loaded with supplements and protein. Sprouts are a snappy source of vitality. They are assimilated into the body rapidly without utilizing a lot of energy.

2. Cinnamon. The flavor cinnamon is useful in directing glucose.

3. Grapefruit. Grapefruit can decrease undesirable cravings and initiates lipolysis, which is the process of burning fat.

4. Ginger. Ginger fortifies weight reduction through fat burning too. Ginger also serves to cool the stomach.

5. Peppermint. The use of peppermint can improve the whole response. Peppermint is invigorating and decreases cravings.

6. Lemon. Lemon contains detoxification chemicals. Lemon performs lipolysis and helps in stifling.

7. Nuts. Nuts are a superb source of protein. Protein gives you a feeling of fullness. Eat lots of unsalted nuts.

8. Chia seeds. Eating chia seeds in yogurt or oats is an excellent way of adding protein and omegas to your eating routine. Chia seeds manage hydration in your body and are loaded with protein and contain each of the three omegas.

9. Greens. Dull green verdant vegetables are superb sources of minerals and vitamins. They help in supplying your blood with the supplements required for vitality and also helps digestive system.

10. Organic products. Crisp organic products are cleansing to the body systems and give you vitality. Natural products are great nibbles that can fight off cravings and help to give you a feeling of fullness.

The best foods for weight reduction work even better when supplemented with every day exercise. Activity burns fat cells and discharges hormones that make you feel good. Increased vitality and weight reduction will be the consequence of practicing and eating right.

Spirulina is a small blue-green algae with an exceptionally rich mix of supplements. This single cell life form has the highest photosynthetic transformation rate (the mechanism by which plants make their own particular nutrients using sunlight) in the plant kingdom.

Indeed, the United Nation's FAO has declared this vitality giving super nourishment as "the best food for tomorrow", which is not shocking considering that 1 gram of spirulina has the same nutritious content as 1 kilogram of vegetables.

Spirulina has been known for a considerable length of time in numerous parts of the world for its excellent wellbeing and medical advantages. Both the Aztecs of Mexico and the Mayas of Central America valued spirulina as a wholesome supplement. Late exploratory studies have demonstrated that no other plant has such high nutritional quality. This miracle foodstuff is extremely rich in proteins (60%-70%) in addition to vitamins and minerals.

It contains a total of sum of 18 amino acids, 9 of which are vital for the human body. It additionally contains a significant mix of vitamins (A, B1, B2, B6, B12, C, E, and H), unsaturated fatty acids, magnesium, potassium, and other components. On account of its fine and delicate cell structure, it is effortlessly processed and immediately acclimatized – it is almost the perfect food for people.

As Spirulina has the most elevated protein content, with around 15 times more protein than steak, it is normally suggested as a nourishment supplement for vegans and sports people. Since it is a highly concentrated supplement, it can be utilized as a part of weight reduction eating regimens and can be taken before dinners reduce the body's craving It does not work in the same manner other craving suppressants because what really does is to bolster the body- through its ease of assimilation – by satisfying the vast majority of the body's overall needs.

Let us now say that you have identified a get-healthy plan and you're attempting to eat well. However, knowing the right nourishments to pick and the ones to keep away from can be another mindset altogether. For instance, a certain brand may boast having low fat but may on the other hand contain very high sugar levels. Also, what may appear like a beneficial meal may be stacked with excess salt. You may not have the time to go through all the ingredients or nutritional content of what you eat, which means that you are diverging from your goal of eating healthy by a wide margin without knowing it

There is no single super food that can help you lose pounds super fast, and not all foods are so bad that cannot be enjoyed occasionally. The following is a rundown of miracle nourishments and foods which you should befriend and that will help you to continue in the straight and narrow and help you attain that ideal body.

Wonder nourishments:

Blue berries. We truly ought to send mother mature a note of thanks for these little gentlemen. They are the best nourishments you could ever eat. They are stuffed with vitamins and minerals and are low in calories. They can also help to bring down the danger of cancerous growths and enhance vision. Why not add them to your hotcake blend, or simply scramble a couple on your grain? Those morning chomps of blue berries will truly light up your morning.

Common yogurt. If you discover yourself experiencing digestion issues such as a bloated stomach or even a yeast contamination, eating normal yogurt will work wonders for you. Common yogurt contains calcium, which is fundamental for solid bones and Vitamin B12 for a good healthy stomach. The taste can initially be somewhat hard to get used to straight away but you can make it more attractive by including your favorite organic product if hacked into nibble sized pieces. Include blueberries to realize twofold health benefits.

Oats. These are basic but ideal for individuals out to create a health improvement plan. Eat them in the morning for breakfast and you'll be sure to be full until lunch time - this will help to remove the nibbling associated with cravings, which set back individuals with health improvement objectives.

Foods to avoid from

White bread. For many people, white bread is a staple food. It can be utilized for sandwiches, as burger buns, as toast with breakfast, and in innumerable different ways. Tragically however, it has no dietary worth. Even two or three slices a day can seriously impede your health improvement plan. The best tip for weight reduction is to remove bread of your eating regimen. However, if you cannot truly live without it, then seek wholegrain bread instead of white bread. .

Lager. To the surprise of many, weight issues are not only associated with food only but with drinks such as lager. Lager can contain high calorific values and should not be included as part of a solid eating routine. Liquor contains no supplements. All calories (which are substantial) are readily absorbed in the body and stored away as fat. What's more, a lager can lead to an extended tummy which does not do much to create a positive self-perception for many people!

CHAPTER FIVE:
DIGESTION IN THE STOMACH

Good morning everybody. Our topic today will tell the truth about digestive compounds and other issues related to the stomach. But before we get to that theme we can start with a small joke I read in the internet. It was distributed by the JokeMaster and is titled "Maturity." Here it goes...

Two elderly women had been companions for a long time. Throughout the years they had shared a wide range of exercises and activities. Presently, their exercises had been restricted to meeting a couple times each week to play cards.

One day they were playing cards when one took a look at the other and said, "Now do not get distraught at me....I know we've been companions for a long time....but I just cannot think about your name! I've thought and thought; yet I cannot recollect it. If you do not mind let me know what your name is." Her companion scowled at her. For almost three minutes she simply gazed and frowned at her. At long last she said, "How soon do you have to know?"

With this said, let shall now discuss stomach issues and digestive chemicals. A stomach issue can be a typical digestive issue such as a stoppage/clogging. Clogging is a stomach issue that makes you have a troublesome or rare solid discharge. Your stool could be hard so that it only passes with significant amounts of strain. It may also be the case that after you have solid discharge, you may immediately feeling like having another discharge.

Another stomach issue can be hemorrhoids. Hemorrhoids are swollen veins that are found in the rectum and rear-end. Hemorrhoids can be of three types. They can be interior hemorrhoids, which include the veins inside the rectum. They do not hurt and they drain effortlessly. There are prolapsed hemorrhoids, which manifest as swollen veins extending down until they emerge as a lump outside the rear-end. This sort of hemorrhoids can be gently pushed it back inside. The third type is the outer hemorrhoids, which includes the veins outside the buttocks. When irritated they cause excruciating pain.

Hemorrhoids arise due to the increased weight in the veins of the buttocks and rectum caused by straining or when defecating. Straining is brought about by looseness of the bowels, weight, difficult work and various exercises that cause the veins to strain.

If you need to avoid such stomach problems, it may be worth taking digestive catalyst supplements. Digestive compounds are the ones in charge of separating food in our bodies and converting them to energy..The Absence of digestive chemicals brings about clogging, heftiness and other stomach issues.

If you were to take your digestive system and lay it out on a large flat surface, the intestines would basically resemble a thin tube. The main exemption is your stomach, which would resemble a large pocket. Your stomach is found below your neck (throat).

Just like the intestines, your stomach is covered with solid muscles that perform compressions called peristalsis. Peristalsis moves nourishment around your stomach and fundamentally transforms your stomach into a kind of food processor which breaks food into smaller particles. While this is happening, there are organs in the stomach divider that produce stomach juices. These juices are a mix of catalysts, bodily fluid and hydrochloric acid.

The stomach produces small amounts of a liquid called gastric liquor dehydrogenase. Liquor is an uncommon supplement based on the fact that it can be assimilated into the circulatory system immediately before being processed. This is the reason why 90% of one serving of liquor is assimilated into the body within 60 minutes.

Stomach juices and other compounds start to process protein and fat by isolating them into essential parts, fatty acids and amino acids. Generally, the assimilation of sugars is not done in the stomach. The stomach juices are acidic to the point that they deactivate amylases, which are the chemicals that separate complex starches into simple sugars. Also, stomach acid can break a few sugars so that a small amount of carbohydrate absorption takes place.

Ultimately, your stomach mixes its contents into a thick soup –like substance called chyme. At the point when a little measure of chyme moves from the stomach into the small digestive tract, the processing of starches resumes. Your body then starts to concentrate supplements from the nourishment.

Move around additional

Normal day to day movements utilizes energy. Create opportunities to get up and move around intermittently. For example, you can get up from your work stroll down the foyer or office to converse with an associate or colleague instead of sending messages by email or telephone. Use the stairs rather than a lift. If using the lift, stroll about inside if there is space. Try to walk to some destination during meal breaks. If you are at home sitting in front of the TV, get up and move around and about periodically. When you using a car look for a place to park some distance from your destination so that you may walk. On overall, change the way of thinking regarding practice and look for opportunities to expend energy whenever possible.

Eliminate Bread

Many of us eats significant amounts of bread. For many, it forms an integral part of their staple foods. – a toast in the morning, sandwich at lunch, franks or ground sirloin sandwiches for snacks or dinners, etc. This bread, especially white bread, contains a great deal of calories. Unless you we are moving about and practicing sufficiently, you will put on weight. Truth be told, bread is one of the worst culprits when it comes to adding to stomach fat. If you need to loose stomach fat, eliminate bread. Do some research and find alternatives to bread – this new alternative will be worth the trouble of finding it. Further, changing the type of bread could be of help. In this regard, note that there is a difference between bread and wheat. Bread is a product refined from wheat.

Eat More Protein

The body utilizes more energy processing protein than it does processing starch. When your body is very still, for example, when you are sitting, your body is working harder to separate the protein. This helps counter the calories and gives you energy. Thus, you do not have to top up with more starches, which can add to stomach fat. You can get protein from incline meat and eggs. Nuts are likewise a decent wellspring of protein but they are extremely thick and have some unhealthy substances, so you need not consume them in very large quantities.

Your digestive framework comprises of numerous parts. Among them is the throat, stomach, and internal organs, tubular structures, through which food and waste items pass and where food processing occurs. Two expansive organs, the liver and the pancreas, produce a portion of the chemicals and different substances required for assimilation. Your gallbladder, an empty organ found simply under your liver, stores bile produced by the liver.

The food you eat is impelled through your digestive tract by strong constrictions that generally are programmed. The processing of the food intake changes it into a shape that is ultimately assimilated into retained into your circulatory system. After the supplements are assimilated, your digestive tract removes undesirable material.

Assimilation starts when you bite your food. The food is broken into smaller pieces by your teeth and at the same time blended with saliva secreted by the salivary organs. Saliva contains a protein called ptyalin that begins to convert starch into sugars.

Chewing reduces food intake to a soft consistency. When you swallow, the food is moved into the back part of your throat, past the opening of the voice box, and into the upper part of your throat. Nourishment is kept from entering your larynx by a fold of delicate tissue that closes as food goes into the throat. If the epiglottis fails to close totally, minor choking and/or a bout of intense coughing results.

The dividers of your stomach comprise of different layers of strong muscles. These muscles, through their mechanical actions cause the stomach to break down the food into smaller pieces while gastric juices fabricated by the organs that line your stomach blend with the food particles. These juices contain pepsin, a digestive compound that starts to separate proteins in the blend, and hydrochloric acid, which provides the correct environment for pepsin to work.

Although the stomach is helpful, it is not the most important organ when it comes to ensuing food assimilation.. Only a small quantity food substances such as liquor, simple sugars, and a few medicines are held in the stomach.

There is a fragile balance between in the stomach between the acid created by its organs and the resistance of your stomach's protective covering to that acid. If this balance is broken and the stomach lining is exposed, the outcome is harmful leading to peptic ulcer gastritis, etc.

Food intake leads to two states in the stomach. The upper segment of your stomach contracts, pushing the more fluid material into your small digestive tract. The less fluid or solid food leaves later, principally by the activity of the muscles in the lower part of your stomach. The partly processed food, chyme, goes through the pyloric trench into the first partition of your small digestive system, the duodenum.

The term digest means to separate or crumble. With this definition, digestion ceases when consumed meals are broken down into components that are suitable for assimilation into our whole body. The greater part of the process of digestion takes place in our digestive or gastrointestinal tract.

The digestive tract is a tube 22 to 28 feet long. As food travels down the digestive tract, it influences all parts of the body.

The point where a substance crosses the cell lining in the digestive tract and is circulated to various parts of the body is referred to as absorption.

The teeth, alongside the musculature from the mouth, stomach area, and small digestive system, have the capacity to granulate, rub, and blend food with digestive juices. Simultaneously, the solid coating of our digestive tract serves to push the digestive blend forward.

Digestion involves the processing of digestive compounds, which will convert enormous and complex foods atoms into simpler substances suitable for absorption. Proteins, starches, and lipids should be split into simpler particles for ingestion.

Bile is essential in digestion and osmosis of lipid components. The stomach area, spanning not more than one foot across, acts like a store for ingested food. The volume of our belly is reliant on the amount of food contained therein. An empty gut may occupy only one to three ounces of space but when full (50 to 75 milliliters) can increase in volume to occupy a few quarts. The stomach is a solid organ. It agitates foods and blends it with stomach fluid. The stomach contains hydrochloric acid (HCl), which makes the midsection an acidic environment (pH 1.5 to 2.5).

A protein digesting catalyst is usually found in stomach juices. This catalyst together with the acidic environment begins the process of protein digestion.

Throughout the day, our stomach may produce around 2 to 3 quarts (around a few liters) of stomach fluid. Past protein digestion, the acidic stomach fluid kills most microscopic organisms in food consumed. The mid-region is fixed at every closure by tight solid fenced in areas known as sphincter muscles.

This keeps acidic juices from entering the throat at one situation and empowers separation in the middle of the stomach. If by chance the mid-section fluid refluxes into the throat, it creates a burning sensation generally alluded to as reflux manifestations.

This is the reason why indigestion is routinely treated with stomach settling agents since they endeavor to neutralize the acid inside the stomach. There are different medicines which can be used to reduce the acidity in the belly.

The stomach is a part of the digestive system.. Food moves from the mouth to the stomach by means of the throat. This food, after being chewed is known as bolus, and is prepared for further digestion in the small digestive system.

The food gathers in the stomach where it is stored for some time. In the meantime, the small entrails have pushed the past cluster and passed it to the digestive organ. The bolus is converted into in the partly digested chyme in the stomach and discharged gradually into the duodenum, the foremost part of the small digestive system.

Separating of protein happens in the stomach with the action of the chemical pepsin. Hydrochloric acid in the stomach kills harmful microscopic organisms. The acid is secreted by the parietal cells in the stomach divider. The compound activity of the chemical digests proteins and mechanical stirring activity of the stomach divider separates the food further into smaller particles. Notably, fats, starches, and sugars go through the stomach undigested. These are digested in the small digestive tract.

The stomach is comprised of four sections. These are the cardia, fundus, corpus, and pylorus.

Food reaches the cardia. The esophageal sphincter situated at the intersection of the cardia and the throat keeps stomach acids from going to the to the throat. The fundus is situated at the upper left of the stomach, it serves to store gases discharged during substance breakdown and agitation of food.

The corpus or body is the biggest part of the stomach. It is the place the grinding or mixing takes place. The fourth area, pylorus, is associated with the duodenum. The stomach is divided into four layers; the mucosa, submucosa, muscularisexterna, and serosa.

Although the main part of the assimilation process happens in the small digestive tract, the stomach dividers assimilate substances such as drugs (e.g. for headaches) and amino acids directly. The stomach additionally has an excellent ability of "tasting" food types, for example, fats, glutamates, glucose, sugars, proteins, and fats.

The travel of food substances through the stomach does not follow the order in which it arrived. Small particles of food and water can go through relatively fast. Normally, food can stay in the stomach for up to five hours. However, the aggregate travel time of food through the digestive system changes with synthesis of food nourishment and the a person's health. The stomach's volume is around 45 ml without distension and can hold up to 3 liters of food.

Research conducted previously showed that the more fully processed meats you consume, the greater the chance of getting stomach disease. Such processed meats include bacon, frankfurter, sausage, salami, ham, and smoked or cured meat. This particular research looked at 40 years of studies on the relationship between such meats and stomach malignancy. A portion of the studies analyzed hundreds of individuals.

Processed meat consumption among study members ranged from under 1 gram of processed meat every daily to more than 56 grams. Higher levels of processed meat was associated with increased stomach malignancy risks. Bacon was the main culprit.

Be that as it may, other substances apart from processed meats (which tend to be more acidic) can be included as dangerous.

Those components that can induce carcinogenic state in the stomach or other organs include other acidic foods and beverages, for example,

1) All dairy items that produce lactic acid.

2) All animal foodstuffs that produce nitric, uric, sulphuric and phosphoric acids. This include fish and eggs. .

3) All sugars that produce acetylaldehyde and liquor.

4) All carbonated beverages that contain carbonic acid.

5) Alcoholic drinks that contain the acidic liquor.

6) Black tea contains tanic acid.

7) Coffee that contains acidic caffeine.

8) Chocolate that contains the acids of bromine.

9) Cigarettes that contain the acids of sugar and nicotine.

10) Emotional anxiety produces an overabundance hydrochloric acidic in the stomach.

Cutting edge medicinal science shows that the stomach needs to be acidic with pH of 1.5 to 3.0. This is one of the greatest experimental myths of the 20th 21st centuries. The fact of the matter is this:

1) The stomach is NOT an organ of digestion but an organ of dedication.

2) The principle function that the stomach does is the production of sodium bicarbonate to alkalize the foods and fluids we eat, not digest them.

3) The solid pH of the stomach is no less than 7.2.

4) As the stomach discharges sodium bicarbonate to alkalize the food and fluids we eat, the pH of the stomach can go up as high as 8.4.

5) To counteract stomach tumors you must strive to maintain a pH of the stomach with basic foods and beverages.

6) The hydrochloric acid deposited in the stomach is not a digestive chemical but rather an acidic waste result of sodium bicarbonate generation by the spread cells of the stomach.

7) The compound association is as per is equation: $NaCl + H_2O + CO_2$ $NaHCO_3 + HCL$ or Sodium Chloride (Salt) + Water + Carbon Dioxide parallels Sodium Bicarbonate + Hydrochloric Acid.

8) The Sodium Bicarbonate made by the spread cells of the stomach ascends to the surface of the stomach to alkalize the foods and fluids we ingest and the hydrochloric acid drops into the gastric pits of the stomach, far from the nourishment and fluids that we eat.

9) Hydrochloric acid is an acidic waste result of sodium bicarbonate and is noxious to the body.

10) Nausea is a state where the body needs the presence of soluble sodium bicarbonate amid times of enthusiastic and/or physical anxiety.

11) The stomach is an alkalizing organ that secures the soluble capability of every other single organ.

12) The stomach is in charge of delivering the sodium bicarbonate discharged by the salivary organs, the pyloric organs, the pancreas, and the nerve bladder.

13) The stomach gets the crude materials needed to make sodium bicarbonate from the blood.

14) Never take supplements or medications that contain hydrochloric acid or various chemicals like, protease, lipase or amylase. They will compromise alkalinity (high pH) of the nutritious trench resulting in health problems.

15) To avoid sickness, indigestion, ulcers and malignant cells, eat, drink and take supplements that are alkalizing (alkaline in nature).

16) Never forget that the human body is soluble by configuration yet acidic by capacity.

As you maintain high alkaline levels, you will enhance the quality and length of your life.

Soon as food enters your mouth and touches the taste buds situated on the surface of your tongue, your salivary organs start discharging saliva. Saliva serves to grease up the food and to predigest cooked starches. In the meantime, your pancreas and small digestive system receive instructions to get ready for the arrival of food and thus prepare to release required amounts of digestive catalysts and minerals required to separate the food into the smaller parts.

One of the most basic reason for digestive inconvenience is gulping down food too rapidly. This dietary pattern portrays uneasiness, eagerness and anxiety. Eating too rapidly diminishes saliva creation in the mouth, which is a notable cause of tooth decay. One of the functions of spit is to keep the mouth and teeth protected against hurtful substances and organisms.

There are different reasons why chewing food well is so fundamental for our wellbeing. As indicated by an interesting investigation at the Gifu University in Japan, chewing enhances memory by diminishing the arrival of anxiety hormones. Attractive reverberation imaging

(MRI) has shown that the hippocampus, which helps control blood levels of anxiety hormones, is empowered by the process of chewing. Thus, the basic demonstration of chewing appropriately brings down both push and anxiety hormones. So chewing your food well can really lessen the levels of uneasiness.

The Japanese analysts likewise found that when teeth were missing or in a condition of deterioration, individuals had a tendency to bite less. This prompted expanded anxiety hormone levels. The conclusion from this study is that good dental wellbeing and the capacity to bite appropriately is critical to safeguarding our memory as we age and in guarding ourselves against the unsafe impacts of anxiety.

After going through the throat, the food enters the stomach. If the food contains carbs (complex sugars and starches as found in vegetables and grains), the salivary catalysts keep on digesting these nourishments for 60 minutes before the stomach starts to emit its gastric juices. If food is swallowed too rapidly, these foods remain for the most part undigested and start to ferment.

Gastric juice is made out of hydrochloric acid, compounds, mineral salts, bodily fluid and water. The activity of the acid kills a large number of the unsafe organisms and parasites that are actually present in meat, fish, dairy items and various foods. The hydrochloric acid additionally separates a percentage of the harmful substances that may go with the food , for example, certain food additives or chemicals. Other catalysts start to work on the proteins that may be in the food. Once soaked with enough acid, the food is constrained in little streams into the duodenum.

The duodenum is an empty jointed tube uniting the stomach to the jejunum, which is the focal point of the three divisions of the small digestive tract. It interacts to the first and smallest part of the small digestive system, and it is the place where most digestion happens. It is known as the top because on an x-ray it look somewhat like a top. Onwards, the duodenum makes a C-turn heading off from the privilege to one side of the stomach area. Bile from the liver and discharges from the pancreas move through the ampulla of Vater to blend with food in the duodenum. The pancreatic juices contain digestive chemicals, minerals and water to help separate starch further. The bile, which is constrained into the duodenum by means of the basic bile pipe, helps in the digestion of fats and proteins. The duodenum takes part in this essential part of the digestive process by discharging particular hormones and digestive juices.

Ayurveda calls the whole movement in this segment of the digestive framework AGNI, or 'digestive fire'. AGNI "cooks" the food with the ultimate goal of making its supplements accessible for cells and tissues at a later stage.

The small digestive tract has an aggregate length of about less 6 meters (18 feet). It is in charge of the retention of supplements, salt and water. Normally, about 9 liters (9.5 quarts) of liquid enter the jejunum (upper piece of the small digestive system) every day, a significant segment of it is made out of digestive juices. The small digestive system assimilates about 7 liters (7.4 quarts), leaving only about just 1.5 to 2 liters to proceed onward to the internal organ. The absorptive capacity of the small digestive system is enabled by a multifaceted cluster of cells lining the inside of its coating (intestinal folds and villi) that assimilate and discharge salts, supplements and water in order to balance the levels of salt and water in the body. In a person, the absorptive capacity is efficient to the point that with a characteristically adjusted eating regimen, more than 95 percent of ingested starches and proteins are retained.

Particular segments of the small digestive tract perform particular capacities. Case in point, the duodenum assumes an important part in facilitating how the stomach removes waste and at what rate bile should be discharged into the digestive tract to improve the digestive process. The duodenum is also an important site for the retention of iron. The jejunum is an important site for the retention of vitamin and folic acid , while the end of the ileum (lower piece of the digestive tract) is the most important site for the assimilation of vitamin B12 and bile salts. The blood takes up each one of the supplements and moves them to the liver for further processing.

The ingested food can be separated into its fundamental component parts and made accessible for the complex metabolic procedures in the body just when AGNI (the digestive flame) is solid. AGNI is powered by bile, without which none of the other digestive juices would be capable of separating food into its constituent elements.

Bile is basic. When food that is mixed with hydrochloric acid enters the small digestive system, it first should be blended with bile before digestive chemicals can follow up on the food. An intestinal pH-estimation of high acidity would square compound discharge and turn into a significant hindrance for the best possible digestion of nutrients. Moreover, with the goal of them being initiated, pancreatic proteins must join with bile before going through the ampulla of Vater. To make this conceivable, the regular bile channel and the pancreatic channel consolidate to form one short pipe before joining the duodenum. The length of bile emission from the liver's bile channels and the gall bladder stay unobstructed by gallstones. Good digestion can be realized only if the ingested food is crisp and wholesome.

The mixture of nutritious food and solid AGNI shapes the perfect organization to help the body make adequate measures of amino acids, fatty acids, minerals, vitamins, glucose, fructose, follow components and other crucial substances accessible to every one of its parts. This, thus, creates solid blood, basic tissues and an energetic body. The nature of the blood and the tissues of the body, including those that make up the skin, generally mirror the state of the liver and the small digestive system.

Stomach spasms are excruciating. There's no other way to put it, other than that they are agonizing annoyances that can be brought on from either over-eating, gas, or digestive issues. If you are a man who often experiences stomach spasms that are food related, then here are a few tips you can put to use to avert stomach issues.

Apart from observing the accompanying standards to avoid digesting problems, one has to chew food properly. . This may appear like an essential and cheesy stride to take, yet it is the one that gives the most advantages to the individuals who use it. Completely chewing your food makes it simpler for it to be digested and assimilated. Once in a while food that is not properly digested may become an important cause of these issues.

The other thing that should be considered is the fact that certain types of food result in the formation of stomach gases.. While you presumably know your own body more than anyone else, make sure to avoid foods that are known to bring about such issues. Regardless of how good the food is, you have to be careful even if you think it tastes great.

It would likewise benefit you to simply exercise some more. While it may appear to be somewhat inappropriate to prescribe exercises to deal with the likelihood of stomach spasms, it is a workable strategy that has been tested since exercising is an effective approach of helping to solve digestive problems. Simply remember that following these steps is a great approach to staying away from the agony of stomach spasms.

Ways in Which Exercise Benefits Digesting Health

We all realize that practice is beneficial for us. It helps us get more fit, gives us more vitality and generally makes us love life. Exercise is also important for digestive wellbeing. Be as it may, we are living in a time where numerous individuals are doing no exercises at all and they are paying for this with bodily weaknesses.

The Functions of the Digestive System

Your absorption is an extremely complex biological process. It comprises of separating nourishment, assimilating supplements into your cells and getting rid of wastes. In the event that any of these key functions breakdown, it won't just influence the digestive framework alone, but your entire body.

Numerous health specialists and nutritionists agree that all illnesses start with a horrible digestive framework. , In response to this, we ought to do everything we can to keep up its wellbeing.

Regrettably, a number of us are living sedentary lives that include practically no physical activity and eating unhealthy diets.

These two tendencies will in the long run harm your digestive framework. Junk foods are loaded with soaked fats that are difficult to process. They block your colon bringing about regular digestive issues, for example, obstruction and irritable intestinal disorder.

How Exercise Can Boost Your Health

Consequently you have to take standard physical exercise as it can truly have different kinds of effects towards enhancing your digestive wellbeing. If you have not practiced before or have you have been dormant for quite a while, then begin to gradually develop your wellness levels step by step levels after some time. It would likewise be judicious to talk with your specialist to begin with, particularly if you have a therapeutic condition.

One of the best activities you can do to kick you off is strolling. Strolling activities have numerous digestive and health advantages. You do not need to run a marathon. Strolling for 10 to 15 minutes a day will have a colossal effect on enhancing your wellbeing.

However, strolling passively is not going to be of much use to you. You need to walk energetically and have your arms swinging and lungs pumping. This will get your blood moving, which is good for your digestive framework.

Yoga Is Great Too

Yoga is another awesome activity for enhancing your assimilation of nutrients and wellbeing. There are particular schedules and activities that put emphasis on the mid-region and these will help to enhance blood flow around your center muscle bunch.

Yoga is additionally a decent approach to eliminate anxiety. Many of us are always worried nowadays because of the busy lives we lead. Encountering a lot of anxiety redirects blood from the digestive framework. This can build acid reflux issues, bloating and inordinate gas.

As should be obvious, joining a consistent activity administration consolidated with a solid eating regimen will enhance your absorption, regardless of the fact that it may be just ten minutes of energetic walk every day.

The human body has more than 600 muscles of different sizes and shapes. They are as threadlike filaments in packs. The mind signals to them to contract which brings about activity. If it happens that the muscles are utilized frequently, they get out of shape and become ineffective. It is through activity that they are invigorated and returned back to great condition.

To keep the heart fit, health experts concur that continuous physical movement suited to various ages and wellbeing is the most ideal approach to keep it fit. This is in opposition to the out-dated conviction that drawn out bed rest helps the debilitated heart. For heart patients recovering from heart problems, it is vital to do slight physical movements, and this has been incorporated in the recuperation program. In the veins, the greasy substances referred to as cholesterol can develop and attach on the vein walls. . Customary activity coupled with a suitable eating routine will help keep down the greasy substances.

Strained muscles can prompt a mental breakdown and it is a sign of anxiety and pressure. For individuals who are hot tempered, have a lot of displeasure, disappointment, stress or other aggravating feelings, activity can give a wholesome alleviation to them. Attempting active strolling or moderate running (or any sort of activity suitable for you) when you are in that state of mind. You will discover that the situation will ease off and you will feel better after you have sweated it out.

A good attitude enhances physical appearance and ensures a good state of the lungs, heart and internal organs. Very well conditioned muscles make it less demanding to sit and stand straight and additionally, strolling with upright body, weight equitably appropriated and muscular strength pulled in. Your back ought to be straight, hips pulled in, knees marginally bowed and rear end tucked under. When you combine exercise with proper foods and abstain from gorging, it will help you reach and keep perfect weight objectives.

There are standards to take before and after you begin your general activity. Ensure that you are sound, and have a physical checkup before beginning a series of standard activity. This applies to individuals who are recovering from illnesses or need to begin working out. It is not prudent to quickly hurry into it because your body will most likely be unable to take it yet. Begin practicing bit by bit and continue at your own pace without trying too hard. Complete every activity accurately with the goal that you fortify your body system securely. Wear free dresses and select an ideal time (best is in the morning) and stick to it consistently on a daily schedule. It requires some serious energy to get once more into shape and do not expect results immediately. Over the long term, with repeated workouts the activities will appear less demanding. You need to keep your courage and do not quit. It is similar to eating, we need to eat regularly.

In case you have had a disease or operation, adopt your doctor's recommendation about the quantity of activity that you ought to do. Quit practicing when you feel exhausted and consult your specialist. If you have been sick for more than a week with minor sickness and no fever, continue your activity routine step by step as you increase the intensity of exercises.

Warm-up activities are those that help you to stay away from over-straining the muscles and increasing the activity of the lungs and heart too quickly. Examples include sit-ups, knee push-ups, toe touching, leg raising, vacillate kicking, arm orbiting, lower leg extending and knee bowing. If you are simply going for energetic strolling, then begin gradually and get the energy as you walk. The best is no less than fifteen minutes a day until you sweat it out or two kilometers of walking.

For the remainder of the day after the morning activity, give yourself positive input, for example, liking yourself and letting yourself know that you are sound. It is one colossal stride to grow a great mental state of mind to soothe stress at work or home. Reward yourself on the grounds that you are qualified for it or carry on with your life lackadaisically. Grinning and chuckling (being jovial) have long been demonstrated as essential fixings to lessen stress. A decent snicker has never hurt anybody and laughter is the best medicine. After a short time, you will be looking buff and pink (sound) and prepared to tackle the world. In this way, do not sit and wait for tomorrow - begin practicing today.

For facial practice, in order to have a tighter and better facial appearance and a healthier gum, wake up no less than fifteen minutes before your designated time and stay in bed doing facial activity. Move your jaws by opening and shutting your mouth hard and move your tongue in and out and sideways. When you wake up, you shall see yourself looking better and fresher. You will help spare your teeth of gum disease.

Running and Your Brain

Running is useful for the psyche. Many of us find peace and tranquility while running since it helps clear your head. Studies have demonstrated that people who take an interest in routine running report that they are more content compared to individuals who do no activity or perform less strenuous activities.

The anxiety that runners feel is associated with the hormones called endorphins that are discharged when you run. This is a phenomenal approach to treat depression or...to simply feel extraordinary!

Coordination

Individuals who keep running on uneven surfaces, for example, climbing stairs or hills find that their coordination increases notwithstanding the numerous different advantages they get from the exercises.

Individuals who run on these surfaces have better control over their body developments because of the concentration needed to remain upright and balanced.

Running Helps Everyone

When you decide to keep running in one of the numerous marathons, (or walks) you get a huge number of medical advantages, as well as that warm feeling of personal gratification form knowing that that you've helped other people with their specific tribulations.

This may sound like a tough cliché, it truly does bring momentous feelings of sentiment, wellbeing and prosperity, and gives you a more uplifting point of view.

A Great Choice for a Healthy Heart

Running is a good exercise for individuals who need to improve their cardiovascular wellbeing. In the course of running, the veins get a huge workout. The heart needs to work harder amid this movement to pump blood throughout the body.

Regular running makes the heart muscles stronger. This has the medical advantage of bringing down circulatory strain and diminishing the danger stroke and other physical problems.

As we age

Notwithstanding improving the heart's wellbeing, different muscles and bones additionally get beneficial outcomes due to running activities. The physical demands on the bones and muscles of the body when a man runs make them stronger too.

Also, people are less inclined to experience a malady, for example, osteoporosis as they age. The debilitation of the bones and muscles as a man ages is not as common in individuals who run compared to those who live sedentary life.

CHAPTER SIX:
10 REASONS YOUR BELLY FAT ISN'T GOING AWAY

If it occurs to you that you are similar to many other over weight individuals on the planet, then you are battling with heftiness issues. For a few individuals, an overabundance belly fat stands out more compared to other body parts. Further, losing the weight here appears to be a challenge. . The truth of the matter is that shedding pounds is not easy, yet it is conceivable with proper planning and arrangements.

Why is Losing Belly Fat So Hard?

Several things contribute to the accumulation of belly fat. These things include: anxiety, hereditary qualities and your eating routine and activity schedules. Of these, maybe the most hard to work with is anxiety-related belly fat. Anxiety must be dealt with to help you lose weight. The primary issue with anxiety is that it promotes the creation of cortical, which has been connected to fat develop around the organs, prompting belly fat accumulation.

Second, hereditary factors contribute a part of the reason for putting on weight. However, your general eating and activity routines can help you beat a characteristic tendency to put on weight effortlessly. Another reason that belly fat is so hard to lose is that stomach activity does little to help lessen the presence of belly fat, and does not generally work to expel the fat from the stomach region. Practices that are focused for stomach zones are for the most part to help construct muscle, not to help lessen fat here.

Can I lose My Belly Fat Quickly?

The straightforward answer is yes. You can lose the weight that has collected in your mid-region as long as you are willing to undertake a couple of huge life improvements. The most critical thing that you can accomplish for your wellbeing is to identify a solid eating regimen and activity routine to help you decrease your general weight, with the goal that there is less weight in your stomach range.

The best activities for losing your belly fat rapidly are oxygen consuming activities that work the entire body, for example, strolling energetically, running or working on a routine shown on DVD or TV. You should practice all the time but also ensure that you are getting the right nourishments in your eating regimen.

Why Not Focus on The Stomach?

The fundamental reason that you shouldn't concentrate on the stomach range to lose belly fat rapidly is because these activities basically do not work. Diminishing your weight must target the entire body, including the food that you eat . Actually, the main approach to lose belly fat rapidly is by having an eating routine of crisp products from the farm (naturally grown foodstuffs), avoiding processed meats and taking a lot of water. In addition to activity, you must have the capacity to get in shape effectively.

Where Do I Begin?

If you discover that you are an anxiety eater, then firstly, what you need to do is to figure out how to deal with your anxiety. You can talk to your specialist, take an anxiety administration class or even start yoga. Secondly, you will need to change the way you eat, and add around thirty minutes to an hour of activity each day to your schedule. With this arrangement, you can lose the belly fat rapidly and keep it away.

Granted, belly fat is ugly. Your garments do not fit right and you may even be consigned to wearing two distinct sizes of attire to make up for your apple-shaped body. Smooth body lines are everybody's wishes. However, you need to know that belly fat not only affects your appearance but your life in general.

Type 2 diabetes and hypertension.

Belly fat "releases" fatty acids into the circulation system, including the liver, the heart and other significant organs. Experimental studies have confirmed that the size of your waist is an incredible pointer to the possibility that you are at risk of building up these ailments. A waist size exceeding 39 inches (or around 1 meter) puts your life in danger.

Being overweight is connected to diabetes in that it causes insulin resistance. Glucose levels ran amok while veins get to be jammed up with glucose and other blocking substances brought by fat. Obstructed blood vessels prompt the emergence coronary illnesses.

Coronary illness and stroke go together as an inseparable unit. Stroke happens when veins in the brain burst (from being blocked). In the event that the brain goes without oxygen for a short a time (about 6 minutes), some parts of the brain involved will stop functioning. Belly fat is specifically connected with blocked veins.

Consider the historical background of your family when deciding your danger factors for coronary illness, stroke and/or diabetes. If your family has these issues, you are likely to have them too. Having additional weight just increases the probability that you will face these problems.

While you may need to decrease your belly fat to look better, you need a greater justification for doing so. The critical justification concerns your health and wellbeing.. What's the purpose of looking great if you can still die from something that is totally preventable? Eliminate chances of coronary illness, stroke and diabetes by trimming the belly fat before these diseases become a personal nightmare. Everybody knows that it's to your own advantage to lose the additional fat from around your belly.

Despite the fact that everybody has a pet name; jam belly, stomach cushions, etc. Whatever you call that layer of belly fat the reality of the situation is that having that overabundance lounging around your midsection is plainly revolting and is perilous to your wellbeing.

Ideally these five reasons will make you reassess where things stand currently stand and help you to act on your situation.

1) Fit Back Into Old Clothes

Wouldn't you want to fit once more into your beloved pair of pants that you haven't worn in God knows for how long ?

That is one of the greatest propelling reasons that I know of. Believe me, I've been there myself.

Furthermore, what better motivation to drop the additional layers of belly fat than to go out on a shopping spree and buy yourself another closet? That is doubtlessly an incredible feeling to shed your current large size and grasp your new, "little" body.

2) Be an Inspiration to Someone Else

For once in your life wouldn't you like to be the individual that a friend or family member or companion can admire as an example of somebody who has taken a decision to turn you're his/her life around to improve things?

You may even have the capacity to persuade somebody to go along with you in the mission or objective to burn the belly fat. They pump up your motivation when required and vice versa. The force of social backing is frequently ignored.

3) Increased Waist Measurement Has a Higher Link to Heart Disease

Research by The American Heart Association shows that overabundance of muscle to fat ratio, particularly when it is situated around the waist, has a enormously contributes to the danger of creating cardiovascular (heart) diseases and stroke. This is not an overstatement.

The startling thing is that they also specify that this is conceivable regardless of the possibility that there are no other dangerous predispositions, for example, smoking, diabetes, and hypertension and so on.

4) Stop Your Arteries from Resembling a McDonalds Thick shake!

Befuddled? Well, look at it along these lines. You know when you get one of those dodgy thick shakes (fortunately my last one was taken as a child) and you cannot suck anything out through the straw regardless of how hard you attempt because the beverage is so thick.

Indeed, that is a situation similar to when your blood attempts to force its way through veins that are all clogged up because of the diets that cause you to put on your belly fat. .

The blood is thick and slow and with very little space to pass through since the vessels are constricted.

The resulting effect is an aggregate blockage and heart failure in light of the fact that the "straw" is completely blocked.

5) You'll Live Longer

For me, the greatest help against getting enormous and becoming another statistic is that I do not need the messenger of death himself to come knocking on my door before I'm prepared. I lost my Dad at 53 as a result of all the above conditions and it is not ideal for somebody to bite the dust in the prime of their life simply because they were too lazy to act.

Also, it must be time to act if your belly fat is at high hazard levels, and that is the place your belly is hanging over your jeans. If you do not make a move now, when do you think you will begin making the move?

It's past the point of no return when you get your tap on the shoulder from death himself.

If that doesn't persuade you, consider not living to walk your little girl down the path and not even getting the opportunity to live sufficiently long to enjoy your grandkids.

Would you like to miss that piece of your later life? It kills me each time I see my little niece and that my Dad didn't live sufficiently long to be around to see her growing up. That shouldn't happen to you and your family either.

If you truly need to get rid of belly fat and get hot abs, you are on the right track. While many individuals worldwide are attempting to lose stomach fat and are spending unlimited hours on various activities to accomplish this outcome, not very many succeed. Why? The reason is their lack of awareness. People simply do not have the slightest idea about the right approach to get flat abs. They do the wrong workouts and they eat in the wrong way.

When you do not have the crudest idea about the right approach to condition your stomach, all the sit-ups on the planet won't provide you any benefit. You will simply be squandering your time in exchange for poor results.

The miserable thing is that all that time and exertion is squandered due to misguided opinions about what is truly important to burn your belly fat and get flat abs.

Here are 3 tips to achieve this:

1. Burn off muscle to fat ratio ratios, not belly fat - One of the fundamental reasons why individuals neglect to get perfect abs is because they make a decent attempt to lose stomach fat and not muscle to fat quotients. The fact of the matter is that you cannot reduce fat from a particular territory on your body alone. You have to take a shot at the overall fat problem and your belly fat will likewise reduce. That is the reason every one of those sit-ups aren't viable. They do not burn muscle to fat quotients. Indeed, they barely do anything by any stretch of the imagination.

2. Make the most of your cardio - Most individuals judge the viability of their cardio workouts by the extent they do it. The genuine estimation ought to be the power level of your cardio and not the extent to which you do it. Running at a fast speed for 20 minutes is a superior workout than doing the circular for 60 minutes. You spare time and burn more calories when you do serious fat burning cardiovascular workouts.

3. Eat to burn fat and feed your muscles - numerous individuals accept that to lose belly fat, you have to radically chop down your calorie utilization. This isn't true. The length of time you take to workout right and eat foods which support your body and not simply make you gather fat will help you burn fat and build your muscles. You ought to eat enough to feel invigorated, alive, and dynamic. Instead of stressing over calories, think more about the sort of foods that you eat. Make your suppers loaded with increased protein, complex carbs, naturally grown products and crisp nourishment rather than pre-made dishes. Not only will you not starve but will also still lose your stomach fat.

This reminds me of a companion of mine whom I discovered had put on some weight and asked him whether he had got his 6 pack yet.

This made me think a bit. He did not wish to get hard abs and was fine with it. To lose your belly fat and get into shape, it must be something you need because it consumes a lot of time. Try not to be too serious about everything or it will quit being fun - you'll require the fun part of it to succeed.

Obviously, for us that have chosen to change our bodies on the grounds that we need it or for restorative reasons, I might want to disclose how to lose your belly fat in a carefully planned and sound way.

Burning fat is something your body is great at doing. However, to do it, you cannot continue letting it fluctuate uncontrollably. To lose your belly fat you need to get your dietary patterns under control and set up your workout in a way that will constrain your body to burn your vitality and the additional fat too.

Many people think they have to do numerous crunches to reduce their tummy and make their abs show. This is really far from reality. Why do you see young men and young ladies in every business doing crunches then? Basically, the answer is to exhibit what awesome looking abs they have and to allure you to purchase their item to get like that, since it clearly needs you to work at it!

The most effective method to lose your belly fat is not about crunches, trust me! The most ideal approach to do it is by pushing your body to work harder. Some do it by running, some by swimming or if you are like me, working out at the exercise center to lose your belly fat.

To begin with, I might want to recommend that you must prepare your entire body when you workout at the exercise center. In any case, the key muscles to concentrate on are your legs and your back. Why?

Because they are the biggest muscle mass a person and they need the most energy for workouts. Have you seen what number of people at the exercise center avoid exercising their legs? Perhaps they do not give much thought to this.

However, the end result of avoiding leg exercises is that their legs will really contrast with the rest of their bodies.

In any case, by meeting expectations with your biggest muscles you won't just prepare your biggest muscles, yet you will likewise expend more energy in the process and thus driving your body to burn more fat.

However, bear in mind that you should eat well . Step by step instructions on losing your belly fat speak the truth. These include cutting off your supply of junk food and the additional fat your body does not require. .

There are a few known eating regimen strategies for that. However, make certain to pick one that suits you or you would likely become weary of it and experience difficulties abiding by it after achieving your objective.

So which is the best approach to lose belly fat? Well the fractional response to that is to prepare like damnation! Then again, the other part of the answer is to ensure that your preparation is successful. This is the reason I have incorporated a solitary hard-hitting activity for you to actualize into your own particular workouts, keeping in mind the end goal so as to get the outcomes you need the most. Read on if I have succeeded in getting your attention.

Lose Your Belly Fat With One Exercise!

As an experienced and molding expert, I can tell that the most outstanding among the most hard-hitting activities that you can to do are iron weight swings. At this point you may be, to some degree, acquainted with the old iron weight and therefore understand that this is one intense quality and molding gadget that will give you out a fit solid body. One of the base lifts of the portable weight is the swing lift. This single lift is especially useful in helping you to lose your belly fat and get you a flat stomach and trim waistline.

The truth of the matter is that if you hope to lose any fat you have look for opportunities to accelerate your body's metabolic rate. This is done most viably by opting for lifts and activities that promptly raise your level of saw effort to bring you to the point where you start to sweat and inhale hard . This is the best way for you to realize any considerable change in your gut as far as fitness is concerned.

This is the very reason I needed to acquaint you with the portable weight swing. This single lift is constantly changing and it includes more than 80% of your body's aggregate exertion with a specific end goal to force it off. If you are going to take part in multi-joint activities to rapidly raise your level of success then iron weight swings are the best to consider as your companions. . This lift requires you to swing the portable weight from between your legs up to the midsection level forward and backward like a pendulum. Keeping in mind the end goal of doing this, you have got the opportunity to use your hips and knees by placing them in a steady condition of flexion and augmentation so as to make the force and energy to swing the chime. This is not just a gigantic activity for aggregate body quality, yet it does afford you cardiovascular wellness too.

If you haven't effectively begun to incorporate the iron weight swings into your own quality and wellness routine, then you are slowing down your advancement. Please do not take the time to think more about this by getting to whatever is left of my articles on the subject for nothing. Keep in mind that anybody can prepare hard, but its best to prepare shrewdly! Is it accurate to say that you are one of the large numbers of individuals that continually battle to lose belly fat? The belly district can be a difficult spot to shed undesirable pounds. The reason being, it has a tendency to be the last place that sheds its fat. We burn fat as we work out, yet regularly the weight will fall off in a few unique zones before it starts to show in the stomach district. This can be baffling to those of us who are for the most part concerned with taking care of our stomach region. Here are a couple of things you ought to be mindful of when attempting to dissolve away your belly fat.

Detoxifying our Systems!

I cannot emphasize enough that it is very important to detoxify your system. This is critical for weight reduction, as well as for wellbeing and prosperity.. Our bodies are overwhelmed by unsafe poisons from the food we eat and the air we breath . If we do not flush these polluting influences out, it can be very difficult to shed pounds. Numerous individuals have neglected fitness on the grounds that their bodies are not working well because of these poisons. This is a very significant variable that people either ignore or are uninformed about. Some extremely viable systems for detoxification are body wraps and fiber supplements.

Try and get a carrot or celery stick rather than a treat, because you may have just eaten at McDonald's the previous week. It's additionally essential to get some activity a couple of times each week. Go out for an energetic walk, run, or bicycle ride for 30 minutes at least 3 times a week. What's more, quality preparations can be extremely valuable when attempting to burn that unshakable belly fat. Due to high quality preparation, you can keep on burning fat, hours after your genuine activity session.

Apply some of these tips to your way of life and results will be seen. Incase you are searching for an approach to target belly fat and other particular areas of your body, I prescribe fat burning body wraps. This is a genuinely new item that has been demonstrated to work wonders. If you are keen on looking at it, I will provide some information. .

You are prone to expand your belly fat if you do not get satisfactory rest. There are a few reasons which may prevent you from getting adequate rest. For instance, you may be a compulsive worker, getting ready for an exam, the TV, undertaking late night activities, focused on some other activity, etc. Whatever it is, such activities affect the way you operate since you cannot get satisfactory levels of rest.

As indicated by a study, individuals who get a normal rest of six hours for every night are 27% more prone to put on weight than the individuals who get 7-9 hours of rest consistently, while the individuals who rest for a normal duration of 5 hours are 73% more inclined to be overweight than 8-hour sleepers.

The individuals who stay alert until the late night likewise, have a tendency of wasting much of their time as they take rest from their work. Surprisingly, young men in high school have a tendency to pick up belly fat compared to their female companions due to lack of adequate rest. One reason behind this is most likely because young ladies can metabolically handle their anxiety better than young men.

It has been found that the less you rest the more fat you have a tendency to pick up. Conversely, with adequate rest, you do not develop fat. As the specialists, would have it, elevated amounts of rest shield a person from amassing more fat.

Incase you do not get adequate rest, you feel tired all the time and do not, , feel the need to work or do some other activity. As mentioned before, the more you stay awake, the more you have a tendency to eat.

Research has found that, all things considered, frequent five-hour sleepers have 15% more ghrelin than the individuals who rest for 8 hours. Still, there are a few special cases also.

Some fascinating perceptions

As indicated by Dr. Neil Stanley of the British Sleep Society, the previous British Prime Minister Margaret Thatcher rested just four hours every day. . The same was the situation with Hitler and Napoleon. None of these persons was fat. Sir Winston Churchill for instance, would snooze for just two hours towards the evening and did not rest much from that point. He had a fat body. Old Indian yogis were exemptions to these perceptions due to their ability to manipulate their bodies through thought. They could obtain the vitality of an 8-hour rest in a matter of minutes. It is said that Napoleon Bonaparte could get all the rest he required when he was on horseback.

If it happens that you have an abundance of fat around your belly and you haven't lost it, you will discover a lot of motivating factors to consider below. Let is review these reasons and see if they ideally inspire you to lose that fat.

1. It puts your life at danger

When you have a lot of belly fat you are in danger of coronary illness, malignancy and diabetes. This is because belly fat overwhelms your inward organs and makes you vulnerable to illness. So, if you have friends and family you have to deal with, this reason ought to inspire you the most.

2. It will alleviate your back agony

If you are battling with back pains, your excessive belly fat may be the reason. . Excessive belly fat places additional strain on your body once again due to the excess weight. By losing excess fat, you will be liberated from back pains. Indeed, even if you do not have back pains right now, excessive belly fat can precipitate it later on.

3. It will expand your confidence

When you can stroll around shirtless again and when you can wear figure-embracing attire with pride, you will quickly feel better about yourself and your confidence will be enhanced..

4. It will make you more appealing

A certain review demonstrated that flat abs is the main appealing body part for both men and ladies. So losing fat will make you more appealing.

5. You will have the capacity to move better

Envision yourself not bearing that additional weight, you will have the capacity to move better and you will feel lighter in light since you do not have excessive fat wearing you down.

6. You will have more vitality

You will have more vitality from the activity and as your tummy is not wearing you down any longer, you will feel significantly more vivacious.

7. It will assuage your gloom or tension

Loss of excessive belly fat will make you feel better about yourself and consequently remove your sadness. Furthermore, if you practice consistently your body discharges a hormone that is called dopamine. Dopamine serves to make you feel great and mitigates your anxiety and tension.

Paunch is a standout amongst the most aggravating parts of one's close to home wellbeing. Fat, when all is said and done can be unsafe for one's wellbeing. This is on account of it turning into a source of undesirable trans fats going through the circulation system and may cause supply route blockages and subsequently, strokes. Stomach fat can likewise make a home suitable for illness by conveying infections and microorganisms. It has similarly been demonstrated that individuals who are corpulent battle with a heap of complexities, for example, despondency, low self-regard and intense fatigue disorder. Fortunately, there are steps you can take to lose gut fat.

When shopping for food, be watchful regarding what you buy. This includes perusing the ingredients to ensure that the calorie levels are adequate. Numerous individuals do not take this pivotal precautionary measure and buy food because of greed and lack. This results in diets that have a high fatty level winding up in the storeroom and eventually on the dinner table.

Another reason for low fat levels is to work out. Some individuals are put off by the control measures included when enlisting at an exercise center or when contracting an individual wellness expert. However, this need not be an obstacle. Simple activities such as running or strolling can suffice. In some cases, even this running can create issues. In such a case, you can basically adopt strolling for short distances instead of driving.

You can also lose extra fat by gathering as much data as possible. They say that information is force and without learning, many tumble off the edge. Girding yourself with information includes basically taking the responsibility to find out more about the reasons why stomach fat collects in the body. Furthermore, joining online gatherings, where individuals who are burdened by the same condition may be beneficial.

If you or your family are experiencing a weight issue then you are not the only one. You are additionally not vanquished! Weight reduction for a healthier way of life can be accomplished by anybody with the right motivation.

One of the reasons why individuals neglect to dispose of their abdominal fat once and for all is on the grounds that they expect diverse results while doing the same thing constantly. If you refuse to dispose off your stomach fat by slimming down, then you have to take a stab at something else. However, for unknown reasons, individuals simply go on another unhealthy eating routine, then come up short once more.

The most effective method to dispose off your stomach fat

If you need to realize different results, then you need to attempt diverse things. It borders on insanity to do the same thing and expect different results. Also, every time you fail you gain more experience since you learn a that a particular technique does not work. Each endeavor to lose fat gives you some sort of an outcome and how you translate these outcomes help you how quickly you will accomplish your objective.

You simply need to eat a little less and exercise some more. Finding the appropriate quantity of food you need to eat and the amount of time and opportunity you have to exercise can be hard. Eating less can function well. However it functions admirably just up to a certain point.

Going below that point may turn you body against yourself. Practice does not have such restrictions, so expanding your oxygen consumption and weight training volume is essential.

In any case, excessive exercise mean that you can strain yourself. If your eating routine sucks then regardless of how hard you exercise at the gym or rec center, , then you won't lose stomach fat. The issue is that more often than not individuals are not informed concerning their advancement by any means. They do not measure themselves accurately. For instance, they do not gauge their muscle to fat ratio levels, their calories or keep a preparation journal.

If you are not doing these things, then it is difficult to locate the right adjustment of nourishment and activity. The more you measure your progress, the more information you get, (both positive and negative), and this means you get the capacity to make more important choices.

How can you stay so thin? How can you get a flat stomach? These are among the most frequent questions I get constantly. Well, there are no insider facts... the answers are in the eating routine and standard activity schedules which I will recommend to you. For individuals who are searching for a quick approach to lose paunch fat, remember there isn't a quick path without surgeries or unreasonable items. In fact, losing paunch fat can be a long process that requires responsibility and consistent practices. You may not see results immediately, but just assume your body is experiencing change. In a matter of time, that gut fat will liquefy away. Let us begin with the tips.

1. Begin with the right attitude

If you are expecting to succeed, ensure you have the right attitude. If you want to succeed, you must have the right outlook. You must set objectives to lose midsection fat. . You need to believe that you can lose the midsection fat. You also need to imagine yourself thin once more. Further, imagine that you have officially accomplished your objectives.

2. Set SMART objectives

Savvy is an acronym that stands for the different characteristics an objective ought to have to guarantee the most success. Objectives should also have the below characteristics:

Particular

Quantifiable (important, motivational)

Achievable (feasible, activity arranged)

Practical (applicable, sensible, results-arranged)

Auspicious

Objective setting is vital and setting SMART objectives helps to support your possibilities of progress. An illustration of a SMART objective may be:

Today is January 1, 2013, and I will lose 5 pounds in a month by Feb 1, 2013... by eating solid and by taking a daily exercise routine in the rec center (or at home), so that I can be sound, fit, have the capacity to fit in my wedding dress, be able to wear my swimming outfit or wear a topless outfit while I am out of town to the Bahamas (find those hot catches and continue squeezing them!).

3. Make an Action Plan & Take Action!

After you have set your objectives on the amount of weight, inches or calories you'd like to lose, make an activity arrangement enumerating your eating regimen and workout schedules. For individuals who cannot manage the cost of a rec center or afford a fitness coach, I prescribe taking this course.

Presently make a move!

The bad news is that it will require a significant investment to lose stomach fat and those extra layers. The good news is that we all realize that it's conceivable and it's feasible. You just have to focus on your objectives and finish. Stop giving yourself excuses that you cannot do it, it's too hard, or you do not have time. The truth is, if you need it badly, nothing can prevent you from accomplishing your objectives. For individuals who say they do not have time, that is just but a weak a reason. Reduce your TV time and organize your time, you will be astounded at how much more you can accomplish in a day.

4. Out with the Junk and in with solid nutritious foods

Dispose off the junk food!

Junk food contains high sugar substances which are high in immersed fat and calories and have little (if any) nourishment. The primary concern is, stay far from them if you need a flat stomach.

Eat healthy - my tips on practicing good eating habits

1. Begin the day with Breakfast

2. Eat fat.

I know it sounds odd for me to instruct you to eat fat when our objective is to lose fat. All things considered, I intend to eat "great fats" nourishments that contain monounsaturated and polyunsaturated fats that are useful for your heart, cholesterol, and your general wellbeing. Some of these nourishments include walnuts, salmon, avocados, and so forth.)

3. Incorporate foods which burn fat for you in your eating routine

There are numerous foods demonstrated to help you to get more, healthy nourishment, for example, bean stew, green tea, berries and whole grains.

4. Expend fewer calories and top off with "great carbs" and fiber

"Great carbs" incorporate foods grown naturally.

Beans-Beans of any sort like dark beans, pinto beans, chickpeas, and add them to soups, plates of mixed greens and dishes.

Entire grains-Eat high-fiber oat, cereal, chestnut rice, entire wheat pasta, sweet potatoes, and so on.

5. Stay hydrated! Drink the recommended 8-oz glasses of water daily to get rid of unsafe poisons!

6. Consume less liquor

If you are a substantial consumer, reduced liquor use will help you to lose midsection fat.

7. Eat more but in smaller bits

Begin planning your suppers and attempt to eat around the same time consistently. Likewise, control the size of the meal by utilizing little plates, bowls, and glasses.

Likewise, take a stab at cooking at home all the more regularly.

Cooking your own suppers permits you to control both quantity of supplements/ingredients and what goes into the food. As we all know, eateries and take-aways usually contain more sodium, fat and calories than home cooked suppers.

3. Exercise schedules

1. Practice in Bursts

Specialists say that in case you are attempting to dispose off gut fat and level your abs, a standout amongst the best systems is interim preparations. Interim preparation comprises of workouts that constitute of bursts of extreme exercises followed with lighter exercises or recuperation.

Here's an awesome interim activity routine you could attempt -(Cardio Blaster).

Step by step instructions to do it:

- Warm up for 15 minutes.

- Then run, bicycle or column for 3 minutes at 90 to 95 percent of your most highest heart rate (ought to feel like 8.5 or 9 on a size of 1 to 10). Take 3 minutes of dynamic recuperation (regardless of whether you're moving, however at a simple pace) and rehash the 3 on- 3 off routine again 3 to 4 more times.

- Finish with a 10-moment chill off.

2. The Plank

To condition the abs underneath your gut fat, you can do the board exercise, which drives you to utilize your abs to hold your body in one position for a broadened period of time. There is a couple of varieties of the board exercise. You can search on various varieties online by typing "board work outs" on YouTube.

CHAPTER SEVEN: VOMITING AND DIARRHEA

Indications of sickness, spewing and a running stomach are brought about by infections. These ailments are for the most part self-constraining. This means the side effects will in the long run disappear by themselves within a couple of days. Periodically, these infections may likewise bring about body throbs, migraines and fever.

Here are a couple of tips for managing these conditions. If it happens that you are experiencing sickness and spewing:

• Do not take beverage or food anything if you are regurgitating often. When your stomach begins to settle, drink some reasonable fluids, for example, water, tea, ice pops, gelatin or sports drinks. Try not to consume any liquor.

• If you feel better in the wake of consuming these fluids, try to devour bigger portions at shorter intervals. The idea is to recharge the fluids that have been lost due to retching.

• If your body is enduring the fluids well, and you have not retched for more than 8 hours, attempt a BRAT diet. That is Bananas, Rice, Applesauce and Toast. Try not to have any jam, spread or sauce. In case you feel your stomach can deal with it, attempt some plain bagels, prepared potatoes or salted wafers. Try not to have any cream soups, plates of mixed greens, vegetables or meats.

• If your stomach holds up well on the BRAT diet for at least 24 hours, you can then gradually begin on a consistent eating regimen. Avoid any seared foodstuffs and dairy products for at least 24hours.

• You can also try certain measures to avoid queasiness such as OTC medicines for 6 to 8 hours as needed to help manage the sickness. If there should arise an occurrence of side effects, for example, throbs or fever, attempt acetaminophen.

In Case of Diarrhea Symptoms:

• Follow a reasonable fluid eating routine until the continuous watery stools cease. . Periodically, caffeine and sugar may compound the looseness of the bowels.

• As the recurrence of the stools decreases, attempt the BRAT diet.

VAs soon as the stool gets firmer, you can gradually begin with a consistent eating regimen.

• Avoid high fiber nourishments like entire grains, plates of mixed greens and wheat for a couple more days and stay away from dairy products too.

• You can attempt some OTC hostile to loose bowels prescriptions.

If there should be an occurrence of sickness, retching and looseness of the bowels, and if the indications do not ease within 24-48 hours, look for restorative help. See a specialist if you are experiencing the dizziness and general weaknesses.. If you are not able to endure any liquids for over 12 hours or if there is blood in the stool or regurgitation, see a specialist immediately . The same applies if these indications are joined by a high fever that does not subside.

It may appear that certain ailments occur due to specific seasons for instance, similar to roughage fever in the spring and fall or colds and flu in winter. Undoubtedly, most ailments that have as their manifestations; queasiness, spewing and the runs are generally infections that one can catch at any given time. By knowing the causes of this three side effects, you will have the capacity to prevent them form happening by taking some extremely basic safeguards.

Regular Symptoms

Whenever an individual is under the weather, regardless of the fact that they may be feeling only slightly ill, as a general rule, they will be having the same side effects as somebody experiencing food poisoning , stomach influenza or even some unfavorably susceptible responses. There are a few individuals who may not fall sick throughout the year. However, change of environment through travel may make them fall sick. Likewise, as already said, the greater part of these cases are viral based, brought about by normal microscopic organisms and infections that can strike suddenly regardless of what time of the year it is.

While the vast majority of these diseases have the same main three side effects; queasiness, regurgitation and loose bowels, you might similarly experience a degree of the following symptoms contingent upon the seriousness of your sickness: stomach pains, cerebral pains, and even dazedness. Should any of these indications manifest, we suggest that you look for restorative guidance at the earliest opportunity. Disregarding manifestations like these for too long time lead to dehydration or some more serious effects. .

Basic Causes

The most widely recognized viral contamination that can strike at any minute is known as gastroenteritis, or stomach influenza. It has every one of the signs of basic influenza. However, one specific side effect that is more harmful with this condition is the looseness of the bowels. Looseness of the bowels occurs when the guts push the stool in your body out before the water in it can be fully reabsorbed. When this happens, you will discharge watery stool continually often accompanied by a fever, spewing, stomach problems and queasiness.

During certain seasons, particularly in summer, the possibility of you taking in poisoned food or some other disease caused by microbes due to increased water intake. For instance, we swim more, drink more, and eat more things than we regularly do exclude in our eating routine. One specific bacterium, the E. coli microscopic organisms, is particularly dynamic amid this season of year. Anybody harboring the microorganisms in the hair or body can transmit them easily, particularly if they have handled fecal matter recently for example, changing an infant's diaper. Most flare-ups revolve around open swimming pools in the U.S and consumption of unfiltered or untreated water in other nations.

Treatment choices

The reality of the situation is that if you catch stomach influenza or some other viral or bacterial based disease, there is no genuine course of treatment that should be possible for you other than keeping you hydrated and on as flat an eating regimen as could be allowed to give your stomach time to recuperate. Truth be told, there are a ton of over-the-counter solutions and anti-toxins that can aggravate your condition rather than better it. It is better to talk to your doctor for guidelines on the best treatment.

Fluids are critical during this time. Since your body has not had room to reabsorb the water from stool, you are losing crucial fluids your body needs to get by with each development. It is suggested that suckle on ice chips or consume small amounts of water or rehydrate.

The BRAT diet

Simply, the best eating routine for recuperating from sickness, spewing and looseness of the bowels is the BRAT diet: Bananas, Rice, Applesauce, and Toast. This eating routine won't upset your stomach but instead keeps the proteins and other nutrients you need at hand and also helps to decrease stomach acidity. In case it is a youngster who is affected, bear in mind that what is useful for a grown-up may not be useful for a kid. So, check with your pediatrician first. Avoid dairy, singed, fiery and citrus nourishments for some time. Avoid caffeine or liquor.

If you encounter retching and the runs on vacation, you could be experiencing Salmonella or E-coli contamination.

Occasional food poisoning is no joke. It can ruin your, journey and also force you to incur costly medical expenses. If you are staying in a lodging and you think your sickness is connected to poor standards of cleanliness at the resort, you can make a case with an individual harm specialist when you come back to the UK.

During any occasion, never eat which is undercooked, especially chicken or pork. If you are staying in an inn, guarantee that food is cooked fresh and well preserved at the right temperatures. Plates of mixed greens ought to be preserved in ice when served while hot food should be sizzling when served.

Occasional grills can likewise bring about food poisoning if meats, for example, chicken and burgers are not cooked completely.

If you are unsure of the levels of cleanliness at your vacation inn, you ought to raise an issue with the management. If you make a written complaint keep a duplicate of anything you sign which will help guarantee payment when you come back to the UK. If other visitors have become sick with similar side effects to yours, take their contacts for future reference in case you plan to confront the inn/lodge administrator.

All inn administrators have an obligation not to expose holiday makers to Salmonella or harmful E-coli in Egypt, Turkey, Tunisia, the Dominican Republic, Spain or at any destination throughout the world. If you have endured ailment in light of the carelessness of hotel/inn/lodge administration/management or the lodging, then you are well within your rights to make a case.

Whether you have endured mild symptoms of holiday ailment or genuine heaving and looseness of the bowels, you ought to look for critical therapeutic help since Salmonella and E. coli can bring about ailment if they go untreated. Lack of hydration is one of the greatest effects of food poisoning. If you lose a large volume of fluids, you may require treatment and an intravenous drip for rehydration.

Kids, pregnant ladies, and individuals with compromised health systems are more prone to suffer from the impacts of Salmonella, E-coli and other causes of food contamination . If infected, you need to you see a specialist as soon as possible. It is additionally recommended, that even after an examination with your GP, when you come back to the UK, you must ensure that you are still not carrying the disease even if you are feeling well.

Food handlers, pose the danger of transmitting Salmonella to customers and partners if they are not healed of the malady before they return to work.

What is nourishment harming?

Nourishment harming is an intense disease that is created by eating tainted or noxious food and poisons delivered by unsafe microscopic organisms. The poisons cause stomach problems and regurgitation. They also cause the small digestive tract to discharge a lot of water that prompts looseness of the bowels. The side effects of food harming typically last under 24 hours.

Be cautious about nourishment propensities in summer. A little misstep can place you in a bad position. From a certain review, it has been recognized that around 81 million individuals are infected from food harming which kills 9000 people.

A notable finding is that it is usually the youngsters who are most affected by food harming. To stay far from this, it is important to be watchful concerning certain things. Food ought to be cooked appropriately and it ought to be refrigerated.

What ought to be done and what ought not to be done :

During summer and for the wellbeing of youngsters, the food ought to be cooked appropriately. Abstain from eating poultry items, meat, fish and eggs.

Utilize the utensils and naturally grown products and ensure that you wash them thoroughly. Diminish the utilization of dairy items and organic product juice. Avoid leaving food in the open and ensure that food in the ice box should be kept below 40 degree F. Abstain from eating packaged food.

Microbes Are Dangerous

Microbes and infections can be found on dairy and poultry items as well . Its preliminary indications are heaving, the runs, pains in the stomach and high fever. After getting the disease, the patient only gets well after meaningful medical attention. If it happens that the disease is not diagnosed quickly, the kidney can be harmed or the individual can lose his/her life.

Issues Caused by High Temperatures

There are two reasons that contribute to increased food harming during summer. First, it is the temperature and dampness in late spring. and secondly the microbes' that spread poisons with quickly. Between 40 and 60 degree Celsius temperature is ideal for their multiplication.

There is a narrow selection certain foods that you can and cannot enjoy when you have diarrhea. Certain edibles are liable to exasperate the framework, by expanding the constrictions of the digestion systems, which you ought to avoid. These foods are bound to intensify the condition, and therefore, avoid from them to bargain viably with Diarrhea.

If you had an attack of Diarrhea, avoid all lactose journal items for quite a while; however you might not have lactose prejudice. The critical lactose containing foods are spread, cheddar, milk, yogurt, frozen yogurt, cheddar. The reason is: Diarrheal conditions for the most part diminish the compound lactase content in the framework. For processing lactose, the process surely needs lactase, which acts on the sugar present in dairy items. If the milk sugar is not processed, you may further experience the ill effects of bloating, spewing, gas, and Diarrhea.

You ought to also abstain from eating high fat substances, which might just increase intestinal compressions. Since your system is as of now in a sharpened condition, high fat substances like fricasseed nourishments, oily things, and rich eatables can just decline the condition.

When you had experienced the onslaught of bowel looseness , you ought to additionally have kept away from simulated sweeteners which are not known to have a purgative impact, but are responsible for increasing gas and bloating in your framework. Till you feel healed of Diarrhea, abstain from taking such things as eating routine pop, without sugar confection, sans sugar gum, sugar substitutes for tea and espresso.

A few vegetables are known for their capacity to expand gas in the intestinal framework, which could exasperate your runs, and henceforth ought to be avoided. These vegetables include beans, broccoli, cauliflower, cabbage, onions and peas.

If you are at the peak of your health, , numerous refreshments containing caffeine or liquor and in addition carbonated beverages do not bring about Diarrhea., However, these things are exclusively equipped for creating aggravation in the GI tract, and in this way it is advisable to avoid these things till you have recouped.

Risky foods

Keep in mind even an extremely solid individual ought to dependably resolve to eat food which has been appropriately washed, securely arranged, and put away in an experimental way. If you consume foods which are not appropriately arranged and put away, it will jeopardize your gastrointestinal tract and cause Diarrhea. Food cleanliness is essential and in this manner you are encouraged to guarantee that you experience the thoroughness of the accompanying safety oriented measures, each time you take nourishment.

Keep in mind to clean your hands, both before planning or eating any food

vegetable and organic product ought to be washed altogether. The area where meals are cooked must be cleaned with a cleanser and boiling point water prior to use and after using the area.

All foods ought to be cooked to a temperature of 160 F.

Subsequent to eating, remains must be instantly refrigerated or solidified.

regulations on certain foods that you can and cannot appreciate when you have Diarrhea. Certain edibles may anger the system, by extending the tightening influences of the assimilation frameworks, and you should stay away from them. These foods are inclined to simply increase the condition, and in this manner keep up a vital separation from them to deal feasibly with Diarrhea.

If you had an attack of Diarrhea, stay away from all lactose containing dairy products for a long time, although on the other hand, you may not be having a lactose bias. The basic lactose containing foods are spread, cheddar, milk, yogurt, solidified yogurt, and cheddar. The reason is: Diarrheal conditions generally decrease the compound lactase content in the system. For processing lactose (the sugar present in dairy foods), the system needs lactase. If the milk sugar is not processed, you may further experience effects such as bloating, retching, gas, and diarrhea.

You should similarly refrain from eating high fat foods, which may very well augment intestinal compressions. Since your system is starting off in a honed condition, high fat substances like fricasseed supports, sleek things, and rich eatables can simply degenerate the condition.

When you experience an attack on your gut , you should avoid recreated sweeteners which are known not to have a laxative effect, besides increasing gas and bloating in your system. Until you feel completely healed of diarrhea, refrain from taking things as pop, sans sugar gum, sugar substitutes for tea and coffee, etc.

A couple of vegetables are known for their ability to create gas in the intestinal structure. These which could worsen your runs and should begotten rid of . These vegetables include beans, broccoli, cauliflower, cabbage, onions and peas.

When in good health, various refreshments containing caffeine, alcohol and moreover carbonated drinks do not cause diarrhea., However, these things are solely prepared for making disturbances in the GI tract, and along these lines it is advisable to avoid these things till you have recovered.

CHAPTER EIGHT:
IS ALCOHOL HARMING YOUR STOMACH?

The fact remains that when you drink liquor it isn't only the calories you should be mindful of. When liquor hits your stomach it is sent to your liver. Your liver then turns it into acetic acid derivation. Acetic acid as a readily available fuel for your body, begins to burn off leaving all other sources of strength inaccessible to your digestive system.

Further, craving for alcohol may increase with time. The more the craving, the more the inconvenience. So you're not just going to stop your body's capacity to produce energy or burn fat when you take a seat to take your meals with your liquor, you're likewise going to need to eat more.

Alcohol also influences your hormonal offset. With an increment in cortisol levels (which sends fat particles specifically to the gut) and a reduction in testosterone levels (permitting you to manufacture muscle with each development) for 20-24 hours, having a beverage or two to calm anxiety doesn't appear like such a smart thought any longer.

Numerous studies have been done on the impacts of consuming large amounts of alcohol for long periods. It has been reliably demonstrated that alcohol abuse does have harmful consequences for your body in the long term. We have recorded five notable outcomes of alcohol consumption and key organs affected.

1. Your Liver

More than 2 million people in the United States experience the ill effects of given types of alcoholic liver illness. The liver detoxifies the alcohol and expels the toxins from your circulatory system, keeping them from accumulating and destroying various cells and organs. In any case, the process of metabolizing the alcohol makes substances that are unsafe to the liver itself. This can prompt:

- Irritation

- Liver scarring

- Liver disappointment

- Death

2. Your Brain

As indicated by the National Institute of Alcohol Abuse and Alcoholism, studies have reliably demonstrated that individuals with a history of alcohol addiction or misuse have smaller, lighter and more contracted brains than others of the same age and sex. This shrinkage in the brain has been shown to result in a few harmful conditions, including:

- Memory loss

- Alcoholic power outages

- Harm to brain cells

- Loss of subjective intuition aptitudes

- Strokes

- Dementia

3. Your Digestive System

Unnecessary drinking originating from alcohol abuse has additionally been shown to harm all parts of the digestive system. . If it happens that you consume alcohol daily, you are at a higher danger of developing digestive system problems such as:

- Unending aggravation of the throat

- Pancreatitis

- Gastritis (aggravation of the stomach)

- Stomach ulcers

- Disease (in throat, mouth, throat, colon and rectum)

4. Your Heart

Another harmful effect of liquor addiction is heart problems and sicknesses. At high addiction levels, alcohol has been demonstrated to interfere with the pumping activity of the heart. It has additionally been connected to various other cardiovascular issues as recorded below.

- Loss of heart's capacity to pulsate appropriately

- Hypertension

- Coronary supply route infection (the main reason for death in Western countries)

- Heart assaults

- Increased danger of stroke

5. Your Immune System

Heavy drinkers experience the ill effects of significantly more irresistible illnesses compared to individuals who drink moderately. One study found that people who abuse alcohol were 15 to 200 times more vulnerable to get tuberculosis than those who do not. In serious cases, the body can stop to precisely separate self from non-self, bringing on the insusceptible framework to really assault your own body.

Notwithstanding the effects of alcohol on wellbeing, the University of Maryland Medical Center warns that liquor abuse can decrease your future by up to 10 to 12 years.

However, there is hope. When alcohol addicts enter rehabilitation, many of the affected vital organs begin to repair themselves and the general strength of the patient progresses.

Going into rehabilitation can be an unnerving, agonizing, and even a risky process. To protect the alcoholic's wellbeing and expand the rate of long term rehabilitation, the first fleeting objective involves detoxification process to help lessen withdrawal symptoms and facilitate the detoxification stage. With this, the following period of restoration can continue with higher chances of success.

Lining your stomach before drinking alcohol: Does it work?

When people talk of having stomach pains, they might really be talking of pains that do not originate in the stomach itself. The phrase stomach agony is used to depict any uneasiness that we feel in the range between the base of the breastbone and the crotch. A large part of this zone may be more precisely termed as the stomach area. In any case, many people use the phrase stomach agony to depict sharp pains in the area as opposed to stomach pains.

In this article, we'll generally avoid discussing reasons for agony that start in the lower midriff – such as crotch pains or a ruptured appendix - and concentrate on pain brought about by anomalies and sicknesses in the area from the base of the ribcage to the area beneath the maritime. That area is also a source of sharp stomach pains and is worth discussing.

Over reveling - Eating an excessive amount of food or eating too quickly may bring about stomach distress. You might likewise eat something you should not: certain meals cause undesired effects in your body or may simply be too difficult for your digestive system to handle.

Stomach infections - obviously, there are interim stomach sicknesses and conditions which may bring about sharp stomach pains. These comprise of stomach infection (ordinarily called "stomach influenza"), which additionally has a tendency to deliver queasiness, spewing and looseness of the bowels.

Gastritis - Gastritis is a problem that is characterized by irritation or removal of a portion of the stomach's lining. Stomach ulcers are a type of gastritis which can bring very sharp and uncomfortable stomach pains.

Indigestion - Most individuals are aware of a condition called acid reflux. This condition, otherwise called indigestion, happens when stomach acid goes past the valve that isolates the stomach from the throat. Since the tissues of the throat are significantly more delicate than stomach coating, some part of the throat is irritated by the acid. This results in a stinging or burning sensation.

Disease - Unfortunately, numerous types of tumor cause no pain until they reach an advanced stage. At a point in time, sharp pain is a typical sign. Stomach disease is relatively uncommon in the United States right now. Those who do are prone to experience sharp stomach pains.

Gallbladder issues - If you suddenly begin to feel sharp stomach pains soon after you having a rich, fatty meals and with elevated cholesterol levels, you may be having a gallbladder problem. Gallbladder issues usually occur when an excessive amount of cholesterol enters the gallbladder so that it experiences difficulty processing it appropriately. A gallbladder problem causes sharp pains and also triggers pains on the sides and the back between the shoulder bones.

Gallstones, another type of gallbladder problem, can bring about extreme distress in the upper stomach area as well.

Liver inconvenience - There are a wide range of sorts of liver issues that cause pain in the stomach territory. These essentially include cirrhosis and hepatitis, which are types of liver irritation. Upper stomach pain is a typical indication of another liver-related condition called ascites. Ascites happens when a liquid aggregates in the stomach. .

Pancreas infection - Pancreatitis is an aggravation of the pancreas and is the main reason for agony in the pancreas. The pancreas helps to regulate the sugar digestive process in the body and when infected, it causes sharp pain in the stomach range.

Spleen - Splenomegaly is the medicinal term for an amplified spleen. When you have splenomegaly, it is typically a sign that there is some other underlying problem or infection. Disease, pallor, or malignancies are among the conceivable reasons. A cracked spleen, which is typically brought about by a blow or some other harm, can cause sharp stomach pains.

Conclusion - This article is written to give you a picture of some conceivable explanations behind sharp stomach pains. Often, such pains vanish before long without treatment. If stomach pains persist for more than one day, then it is advisable to consult your physician.

Strawberries Will Protect Your Stomach from Alcohol

These tough little fruits from the rose family are some of our most basic mending herbs. The name strawberry originates from an old English word meaning "strewn over the ground". Ripe strawberries can give the impression of being strewn over the ground. Fragaria originates from the Latin word for "scent," and virginiana comes "from Virginia." The first recognized species were most likely from the Virginia districts. The vast majority of our local plants were identified and named by European naturalists in the 1600 and 1700s. A demand for such plants and other new opportunities in untamed New World (as America was called during this period) brought numerous pioneers to these shores.

There are maybe twelve types of these low-lying and enduring herbs, with established runners that can cover an entire region. The excellent compound leaves partition into three flyers and have serrated (toothed) edges. The wood strawberry has pointed flyer tips, while the regular or Virginia strawberry has adjusted pamphlet tips. The exemplary white blossoms have five petals covering the inside, which grows and ages into the beefy red natural products, which are not genuine berries, bearing seed-like achenes on the organic product surface. Local to northern mild areas, strawberries will develop in any soil and are broadly appropriated across North America. Field researchers noticed that the wild strawberry was the first plant to colonize the edge of Mount St. Helens, developing in volcanic cinder, after the well of lava cooled down after its ejection in 1980.

A local Indian image of richness and consecrated recharging, the wild forest strawberries are replicated and regarded in wicker bin, wood carvings, quillwork, moose hair weaving, and beadwork outlines. We see our wild strawberry plants, blooms, and organic products imprinted all over, from cradleboards to customary apparel, as it is accepted that they convey uncommon gifts.

Customary employments:

The restorative ethics of these plants were very much investigated by the Indians. In the mid 1600s, Jesuit ministers working among the Huron in southern Canada depicted one of the Huron curing services with clear surprise. Tscondacouane, a visually impaired Huron man, envisioned that it was critical for him to quickly keep in mind the end goal to end a boiling over pandemic among his kin. He fasted for seven days, whereupon the spirits said to him, "We can do nothing more to you, you are connected with us, you must live henceforth as we do, and we must uncover to you our nourishment, which is just clear soup with strawberries". After this the Huron ate dried strawberries amid the winter months all together not to get debilitated. This was additionally the practice among different tribes, as wild strawberries were unbelievably, various hundreds of years back and effortlessly gathered and dried for future utilization, as were cranberries, blueberries, blackberries, and numerous sorts of raspberries.

Roger Williams, living among the Narragansetts in 1643, expounded on the universal wild strawberries, praising their numerous Excellencies. He noticed that they were so productive in a few territories where the Indians had planted them, that there was 'organic product 'enough to fill a decent ship. The French brokers noticed the significance of exchanging certain things for new and dried strawberries with different northern tribes. Most tribes used them as part of teas or decoctions to ease stomach infirmities, spasms, menstrual challenges utilized the mitigating, astringent leaves, and as restorative body washes to calm sunburn, rashes, and other skin aggravations. Strawberry root teas were taken as blood purifiers, diuretics, and digestive guides, and the roots were chewed to mitigate toothaches and sore throats, hacks, and upper respiratory trouble. A few tribes utilized solid leaf decoctions as nerve tonics, to treat kidney and bladder issues, and to cure the runs.

Advanced employments:

Today strawberries are developed as ornamentals, ground covers, for natural needs, and particularly for their eatable organic products. Both crisp foods grown from the ground are high in vitamin C. Strawberry flavorings, vital oils, and quintessence have extraordinary business esteem in everything from dessert and yogurt to shampoos, fragrant healing, home grown healthy skin, and mitigating natural recuperating recipes.

Cutting edge cultivators respect the numerous remedial characteristics of these wild plants. The ready natural products can turn out to be intestinal medicines for a few individuals, and a few people are allergic to strawberry seeds. Strawberry leaf tea is a trusted, gentle guide to absorption and can likewise animate the hunger.

There are numerous extraordinary medical advantages of strawberries, and we are going to examine the advantages for those people who choose to add them to their eating routine.

Phenol cancer prevention agent insurance

Strawberries are known as a rich wellspring of phenols. Anthocyanins in strawberries do not just give wonderful shading to these natural products, but additionally, they serve as cancer prevention agents that ensure cell structure development in the body. Phenols in this natural product ensure that the heart is strong enough to battle against disease and aggravation. Mitigating properties of strawberry incorporate the capacity offered to diminish the phenol cyclooxygenase compounds. Nonsteroidal calming medications like headache medicine or ibuprofen help in clearing agony by blocking chemicals that add to the improvement of aggravation, for example, those happening in osteoarthritis, rheumatoid joint inflammation, asthma, atherosclerosis and tumor. Not at all like the medications that square COX compounds, strawberries do not bring about intestinal degeneration.

Phytonutrients in strawberries guarantee ideal wellbeing

Elagitanin substance of strawberries has been connected with a lower danger of death brought about by malignancy. Individuals who frequently eat strawberries demonstrate a three times lower danger of growth contrasted with others.

Insurance against Rheumatoid Arthritis

Albeit one study demonstrated that high dosages of vitamin C lead to the event of osteoarthritis (the most widely recognized type of joint pain, basic in the elderly), different studies propose that substances rich in vitamin C, for example, strawberries, cushion people from joint pains.

Strawberries - Selecting and Maintaining

1. Pick a hard natural product, with vast, dark dabs and a lovely shading, joined to a green stem

2. Strawberries are exceptionally perishable and require consideration. They can be put away in the fridge a day or two. Try not to abandon it too long at room temperature or in the sun in light of the fact that it will get ruined.

3. To stop them from deteriorating, wash them delicately and after that slice them well. Place them on a solitary line. When solidified, store them in a pack and place them in the cooler. Showering them with a little lemon juice will help them to keep the shading. In the event that they are left in place and not cut in pieces, strawberries will keep a bigger measure of vitamin C.

4. Anthocyanins can be found in both crisp strawberries and in the solidified, however, not prepared items.

Eat protein-rich food when drinking alcohol to protect your stomach

Counting high protein sustenance in your eating routine is one of the approaches to shed pounds. Your body needs to work harder to process and separate the protein. Truth be told, your body can burn calories by simply handling the protein. One of the reasons why a large number of individuals put on weight is because they making up for lost time in the current inclination to eat chiefly starches. If you consider the quantity of dinners that are full of starches, you will recognize what I mean.

Getting the perfect measure of protein is not a careful science, but rather there is by all accounts an accord among nutritionists that8 grams of protein per bodyweight in kilograms is safe. . At the end of the day, reproduce your body weight in kilos by.8 and your weight in pounds by.37. The Harvard School of Public Health says you can get 20-25 percent of day by day calories from protein with no unfriendly health dangers. It does caution those with kidney ailment not to take in more than the suggested sum.

Here are a few nourishments that are great wellsprings of protein and are promptly accessible:

- Meat

- Fish

- Eggs

- Dairy items

- Vegetables

- Seeds and nuts

Meat is high in protein yet incline meat is best to avoid from abundant measures of soaked fats. The meats to search for are incline hamburger, sheep, bison, and chicken. Be mindful so as not to eat any meat essentially on the grounds that it has protein. For instance, a little bacon every once in a while is okay yet you would not have any desire to make it part of your daily diet. Handled meats in wieners and chilly meats like salami and ham and chicken moves ought to be shunned. .

Fish has about the same measure of protein as meat without the immersed fats. Eggs are likewise a decent wellspring of protein and they are anything but difficult to get and simple to cook. They were considered to raise cholesterol levels yet recent research has demonstrated this to be false. Dairy items, for example, drain, yogurt and cheddar provide protein, although they additionally contain soaked fats. Skim milk is fine as is other dairy nourishment, but with some restraint.

Beans are one of the best wellsprings of vegetable protein. While there is some dialog about the benefits of individual assortments in light of the fact that some contain a high rate of starches, there is no debate as to their protein content. Most have around 20 percent protein or better. Beans, for example, kidney, red kidney, pinto, Lima, naval force, incredible northern are all great, economical wellsprings of protein. Shouldn't something be said about the terrible jokes on the impact of beans on your stomach and on the individuals around you? It is genuine they do make twist, so ensure you soak them in water before you cook them.

Seeds and nuts are another wellspring of protein. Notwithstanding that they contain supplements and vitamins. Some of them, similar to flax seed, are little and hard to eat. However, walnuts and almonds are less demanding to handle and can without much of a stretch be incorporated in snacks.

Nature has given us numerous wellsprings of protein as it makes up about a large portion of our body weight and is vital for our bodies   for maintaining a great   shape. One way of maintaining good health is holding weight under control. Eating more protein will help you do this.

A few individuals discover it is truly hard to put on weight. They eat, eat and eat some more, and prepare as hard as could be expected under the circumstances, yet at the same time battle to make the scales climb even a large portion of a pound. So what's the key to putting on muscle in case you're a hard gainer?

 gainers miss the mark in is protein utilization. Calories are critical for muscle development, as you furnish the body with vitality to manufacture the muscle, , it will be for all intents and purposes difficult to fabricate considerable muscle if you are not getting sufficient amounts of protein.

Every protein atom is comprised of twenty amino acids. Amino acids are the building blocks of muscles, and without these, the body is not going to have the capacity to include, or even maintain weight. This is the reason sufficiently expending protein is crucially critical.

So, calories admission and protein utilization appear to be the two regions where hard gainers need to give careful consideration, with a specific end goal to achieving   their objectives. In view of this , the proposed nourishments will be both high in calories, and protein.

Entire Eggs

Entire eggs are a phenomenal nourishment. The yolk has been vilified for a considerable length of time, yet at long last, the restorative calling and the overall population give off an impression of having understood that the yolk contains numerous critical vitamins, minerals, and solid fats, and does not have an antagonistic impact on cholesterol levels. One substantial entire egg conveys around 90 calories, and 8g of protein, contingent upon the size. They're an awesome choice for breakfast for the individuals who cannot stomach meat or fish first thing in the morning, and would prefer not to depend on having a protein shake.

Eggs are likewise to a great degree flexible. They can be bubbled, poached, fricasseed, mixed, cooked as an omelet with included vegetables, cheddar or meat, added to servings of mixed greens and used to raise the protein levels of whatever other meal. They're the perfect nourishment for a hard gainer.

Hamburger

Numerous weight lifters settle on chicken or turkey over red meat; however they're feeling the loss of a trap. Whilst hamburger and chicken both contain around 25 grams of protein for each 100 grams, contingent upon the cut, 90% incline meat gives approximately 165 calories, contrasted with 110 in the same measure of chicken. For a hard gainer, this is a no challenge - hamburger wins come what may. Hamburger is likewise a splendid wellspring of iron, B vitamins, and zinc.

On the off chance that you can, It is preferable to pick grass bolstered and unfenced red meat, instead of meat from industrial facility cultivated creatures. Dairy animals are intended to live off grass, and not the corn that they're encouraged to feed on in the processing plant homesteads. They are likewise permitted to develop at their regular rate, and not pumped with chemicals, so

175

that they can look much healthier. You'll see a gigantic distinction in taste and healthful quality in an unfenced meat.

Sleek Fish

Another important food that enriches one's diet is fish. Once more, I'm interested in referring to the reasons why it harvests up so regularly, as it is a low calorie sustenance. 100 grams of fish provide 120 calories, and 27 grams of protein. The same measure of salmon has 200 calories, and 25 grams of protein. Whilst protein is somewhat brought down, 25 grams for every hundred is still a sensible sum, and as we've stated, - calories also contribute a huge part in muscle development, and so is salmon and trump fish.

Salmon and other sleek fish like mackerel, sardines, anchovies, trout and herring additionally give a lot of fundamental fats, known as omega 3 fats. Devouring a high measure of omega 3 is accepted to lessen a man's danger of coronary illness, support the insusceptible framework, and help ease joint and muscle pain.

Entire Milk

Whilst not actually a nourishment, entire milk gives loads of good quality protein, and also some immersed fat, which is important for managing hormones inside of the body, especially testosterone, which assumes a crucial part in muscle development. The reason I've included it here is because milk is calorie thick, and simple to drink. 100 milliliters of entire milk will give you 68 calories and 3.4 grams of protein. Whilst this doesn't sound like a great deal, it is anything but difficult to have a glass of milk nearby every dinner, and several pints for the duration of the day. Without even realizing it, you can expend an additional 68 grams of protein and 1360 calories, and still have enough of ravenousness for all your nourishment.

CHAPTER NINE:
HOW THE GUT'S "SECOND BRAIN" INFLUENCES MOOD AND WELL-BEING

The early breakouts

Numerous individuals battle with skin breaking, most eminently young people, and those in their youthful years. In any case, it is a certainty that numerous individuals who experience the ill effects of it at a youthful age likewise endure it later on in their grown-up years. Skin inflammation can rise whenever in a man's life.

It is not advisable to ignore skin problems especially when it starts to break. When you are a grown-up, there can be more inconveniences so it's best to zap it when it first develops. Gone untreated for years, skin break out can re-surface as a more propelled skin issue, for example, scarring.

There are a wide range of reasons that contribute to cases of skin break out on somebody's skin. Many people think it is a hereditary condition. It commonly strikes practically everybody at an early stage to some degree or another. Generally speaking, getting it right off the bat will make things less demanding for you.

You ought to go to a dermatologist when you discover that you have serious skin inflammation. They will let you know what pharmaceutical and skin inflammation treatment items are best for what kind of skin you have. Everybody is diverse and in this manner needs different sorts of pharmaceuticals. If you utilize the wrong pharmaceutical with your skin sort, you could exceptionally well see antagonistic impacts.

In today's cutting edge age, there are various sorts of skin inflammation medications running from balms and salves to all the more, top of the line, costly medicines like laser or light evacuation that you can utilize with the help of an expert. In any case, it is exceptionally prescribed that you go for the more secure choices before investing loads of cash and energy into different strategies.

One good thing to remember dodging is when meds rely upon Vitamin A subordinates. Those items could wind up with breakouts rather than clear skin.

Contingent upon your kind of skin, there are medicines out there that will work for you, it's simply a question of being patient and discovering what lives up to expectations for you. Investigate every one of the choices on the table; yet do not be eager at the same time.

Notwithstanding the immense things individuals say in regards to some skin inflammation items, I have found that most skin break out medications basically did not work for me.

Yet, following quite a while of attempting to dispose of my skin break out, I at long last discovered something that had the capacity to totally cure my skin break out in only a couple of weeks.

The discovery of the Second brain

How often have you moved out of bed, looked in the mirror, then turned sideways and simply let out a loud murmur? You attempt to suck it in however it doesn't work. I wager you did only that early today? Possibly it has become relentless for some time now and the occasions have quite recently exacerbated it. Well it's opportunity to burn off that tummy fat and level your stomach. I was doing literally the same thing only a couple of months back. I had an awful injury while playing and consequently, I was laid up for some time doing nothing. I was putting on weight relentlessly and turning out to be more unfit. My conditioned stomach had gone and a layer of fat had moved in and flourished. When I got sufficiently sound to begin playing again I figured it would be gone in a month.... boy was I off base.

You see I'm picking up on 30 now and no spring chicken any longer, and my body doesn't burn the fat off as effectively as it used to, having been pregnant twice doesn't help your tummy muscles out either. So I chose to make a move and dispose of my heavy stomach. I hit the exercise center hard, doing many, many crunches and preparing like an insane person attempting to burn of that tummy fat.... Nothing. Try not to misunderstand me, I showed signs of improvement than I had in quite a while. In any case, that layer of fat just wouldn't move! I was beginning to get discouraged and neurotic about it. I feared running, swimming with my two young men, or setting off to the shoreline. I wouldn't wear garments that were tight around my tummy when I went out, which I used to do all the time with pride. So I began to scan for an answer on the web. I had resolved to dispose of my out of shape stomach.

When I had found a few items that demonstrated to me proper methodologies to burn off gut fat with no sweat, I understood I was turning out badly. You see I've generally played some kind of game and have been dynamic. So I've never had an issue with my body and, in this manner, never needed to burn off a fat tummy. So I recently assumed that setting off to the exercise center would sort it. Well now, I've found it's really less demanding than that.

It's about eating routinely and having controls in place. I figured out how to change the nourishment I ate, and get more products of the soil such as vegetables. Cook things distinctively and remove the slippery snacks. None of this was an issue to me before on the grounds that I was so dynamic. However, I discovered that once your body moves beyond a certain stage, it will never retreat to how it used to be if you bear on like you generally did. I resolved never to eat certain sorts of sustenance after 6pm., This is because the body goes into a resting mode as you rest and doesn't process nourishment in the same way as if it were not at rest.

When I found how to treat my body the right way, I discovered that 30 minutes of preparing at home was all it took to recover my conditioned stomach. 20 minutes of relentless activity in addition to 10 minutes of crunches and leg raises, 4 times each week was all I needed to do. I am currently back on the shoreline and out in my tight garments with my head held high, and you can be as well. Find how to level your tummy as I did, dispose of that gut fat, tone up your stomach and recover your certainty and self-regard.

The autonomic nervous system

The most fundamental units of the autonomic sensory system, the nerve cells transmit signals electrically inside of the phones. However, this happens artificially when signs traverse a hole under one millionth of an inch to another cell, in this manner looking like a refined system of living "wires" responsible for putting on and off the digestive framework at the proper time.

On account of a normal solid individual, autonomic nerves in his mind expand the generation of spit as he chews sustenance amid a lovely supper. Autonomic nerves in the belly expand the movement of the smooth muscle and organs in the stomach and digestion tracts in this way advancing peristalsis. In the wake of staring at the TV, this fulfilled cafe washes up, and gets prepared to hit the sack. While he utilizes the restroom, the autonomic nerves in the pelvic area urge him to poop.

Every one of the nerves effectively included amid this unwinding period emanates from two areas: the base of the noggin and the substantial triangular sacrum bone between the hipbones. This is the 'rest and review framework,' some piece of the autonomic sensory system called parasympathetic nerves.

There is a special case to consider for the unwinding part of the parasympathetic nerves. At the point when a man has the alarm of his life, parasympathetic nerves could animate his gut to poo on the spot making the "frightened" impact.

Then again, when a man awakens late in the morning and spruces up in rush to work, another arrangement of autonomic nerves become dynamic. The thoughtful nerves found between his neck and waist, the lower piece of his back and close by the spine set him up for the unpleasant circumstance expanding the rate of his pulse, expanding the stream of blood to muscles and redirecting blood far from the gastrointestinal tract, in this way putting off his inclination to crap.

Thus the thoughtful nerves fill a gainful need in postponing crap. Individuals, who are focused, are successfully setting off this 'battle or flight framework' and preparing their insides to, in the end, go obstructed.

Despite the fact that the thoughtful and parasympathetic frameworks have inverse activities in their impacts on the digestive organs, they ordinarily work in a corresponding manner to deliver fine control of the body's life-bolster capacities. Generally these two frameworks control automatic body capacities, which incorporates processing. Now and again, the enteric sensory system implanted in the dividers of the stomach and digestion systems is recorded as an extra piece of the autonomic sensory system. It controls digestive development and emissions.

CHAPTER TEN:
HOW DO YOU PROTECT YOUR STOMACH FROM NSAIDS?

NSAIDs stop the Cox proteins in our body from working. They accelerate our body's generation of prostaglandins. Prostaglandins cause the sentiment agony and control body temperature by aggravating your nerve endings. The diminished level of prostaglandins in your body, make NSAIDs simpler to ease pain from conditions like joint inflammation. They additionally help decrease irritation, lower fevers and keep blood from coagulating. At the point when Cox compounds are blocked, pain and ceaseless aggravation is lessened, yet the defensive coating of your stomach is likewise decreased. This can bring about issues, for example, ulcers and draining in your stomach and entrails.

There are different genuine reactions of utilizing NSAIDs drugs.

Case in point:

Yellowing of your skins and eyes.

Essentially weight pick up.

Feel spasms, shivering, and deadness on your muscles.

Blood in pee.

Hypersensitive response: trouble breathing, swelling lips, tongue or face.

Shouldn't something be said about Omega 3 supplements? Is it true that they are recoverable?

Exploration demonstrates that fish oil has positive changes in blood lipids, and a more noteworthy rate of abatement after the 3 years - 72 for each penny contrasted with 31 for every penny in the non-fish oil bunch. It can diminish cardiovascular hazard in RA patients, and that this takes places by means of a few natural pathways. Numerous researcher propose that fish oil could possibly swap drug treatment for some RA patients. One study shows, NSAIDs medication utilization was diminished by 75 for each penny in the fish oil gathering between the beginning and completion of the study, contrasted and 37 for each penny in the non-fish oil bunch. Fish oil is less expensive, a more secure treatment alternative and could likewise serve as a safeguard measure against joint inflammation.

What are NSAID's?

NSAID's, or non-steroidal mitigating medications, are a class of medications, some recommended by specialists and others accessible over the counter, for the treatment of aggravation, gentle to direct agonies, joint inflammation and fevers.

How do they function?

NSAID's work in conjunction with your body's coenzymes, specifically Cox1 and Cox2. Those coenzymes are in charge of discharging prostaglandins, which, , cause pain, aggravation and fever. By taking NSAID's you can restrain this response, hence diminishing the creation of prostaglandins and the pains you are encountering.

What conceivable side influences should I be careful about?

Lamentably, by keeping the prostaglandins from bringing on you fever and pain, you are likewise keeping the coenzyme Cox1 from performing an amazingly important capacity - protecting your stomach. Prostaglandins created by Cox1 are in charge of ensuring that the mucous coating of your stomach remains intact, and in addition supporting your body's generation of platelets, a blood segment instrumental in the blood's capacity to clump. By taking a lot of NSAID's more than an expanded time of time, you are putting yourself at danger for harm to your stomach lining, an ulcer, or uncontrolled death.

In addition to this, NSAID's have other "general" stomach-related symptoms you should be careful about, for example, diminished ravenousness, obstruction, the runs, regurgitating and queasiness.

A Below is a rundown of the most famous NSAID's available and their utilization:

Celebrex - a mitigating sensitivity drug. Accessible by medicine just. Turned out to be moderately ok for the stomach, with a set number of negative symptoms.

Ketorolac - a fairly intense NSAID that operates as an agony blocker. Unreasonable utilization can bring about serious harm to the coating of your stomach.

CHAPTER ELEVEN: STOMACH ULCERS: HOW TO DEAL WITH THIS MENACE

Influencing a huge number of Americans every year, a stomach ulcer is a crude, open wound in the coating of the stomach. Stomach ulcers get their specific name contingent upon the definite area of the ulcer. Case in point, a duodenal or peptic ulcer is a stomach ulcer found in the first foot of small digestion systems past the stomach. A gastric ulcer in situated inside the stomach itself. Albeit duodenal or peptic ulcers are quite often , and it is vital to recollect that gastric or stomach ulcers can be threatening. Close restorative administration is discriminating.

A defensive layer of bodily fluid creating cells keep the stomach from being obliterated by ordinary digestive squeezes and stomach acids. On the other hand, when there is a break in, a bad situation can happen. A stomach ulcer happens when the gastric or intestinal mucosal coating of the stomach is wrecked by hydrochloric acid, a acid which is typically present in the digestive juices of the stomach.

Another reason for ulcers, especially gastric and duodenal ulcers, can be a bacterial disease known as Helicobacter pylori or H. pylori. The helicobacter pylori bacterium may be transmitted from individual to individual through polluted nourishment and water and is treated with anti-infection agents.

One of the significant side effects of a stomach ulcer is pain., This particularly is pain that feels much like a biting or burning pain in the center upper mid-region frequently happening around a few hours after a feast. Frequently this pain is confused for acid reflux or significantly hunger. Pain from a stomach ulcer may stir you during the evening and may be assuaged with nourishment or milk.

Stomach ulcers are treated with remedy quality pharmaceuticals intended to decrease stomach acid, to secure the stomach lining and to treat the H. pylori microscopic organisms, if it is available.

Not all nourishments are useful for the stomach. At the point when the stomach is experiencing ulcers, it is important to realize what the great and terrible nourishments that alleviate stomach ulcers are.

Ulcers are wounds in the coating of the digestive tract. Sorts of ulcers are recognized where they happen. Duodenal ulcers will be ulcers in the duodenum. Ulcers in the stomach are known as gastric ulcers and ulcers in the throat are called esophageal ulcers.

What Causes Stomach Ulcers

There are different reasons for the occurrence of stomach ulcers, yet all are connected to nourishment and acceptable cleanliness. Some time recently, most specialists accepted that ulcers are essentially brought about by anxiety and by eating an excessive amount of acidic nourishments. Yet, that all changed after a research center trial found that a microbe called H. pylori causes the disease in the digestive tract by causing injuries. Acidic sustenance and gastric juices can just irritate the bruises by burning the digestive tract dividers.

Ulcers in the stomach are additionally brought about by some mitigating meds. These medicines are what specialists for the most part provide for patients with joint pain. These can be destructive to the stomach lining., So, if taken for a long duration of time, they can build the foundation for ulcers. Naproxen, ibuprofen and headache medicine are a portion of the known mitigating medications that may trigger stomach ulcers.

Step by step instructions to Treat Ulcers

As specified earlier, stomach ulcers are essentially brought about by contamination. So the essential suggestion that your specialist will give you will be to treat the wounds by murdering the microscopic organisms first. This prescription will keep going for 2 to 3 weeks or until there's no more hint of the microorganisms in your stool. On the other hand, this treatment may not generally be powerful for individuals experiencing different illnesses like diabetes and joint pain.

So to keep away from any intricacy, why not treat stomach ulcers normally?

The Bad Foods

Clearly, you wouldn't have any desire to encounter its side effects. You would prefer not to feel the pain and see blood in your stool. Henceforth, you must avoid from acidic sustenance that may trigger these side effects. Liquor, caffeine, fiery nourishments and high admission of sodium (or salt) can all add to this infirmity. The initial three build the creation of acids in the stomach while sodium can disturb its dividers.

Sodium is contained in salt as well as most meds and vitamin supplements contain sodium at a level superfluous for our bodies. If you are taking some different medicines, you must drink bunches of liquids, particularly unadulterated water to help wipe out exorbitant sodium quick.

What are Stomach ulcers and why they come to be?

Stomach ulcers, otherwise called gastric ulcer or peltic ulcer, is an injury that structures in the coating of the stomach.

Specialists used to suggest that a distressing way of life and a less than adequate eating routine brought about ulcers. Later, it was found that a reeling between digestive liquids (hydrochloric acid and pepsin) brought about ulcers. Today, research demonstrates that most ulcers grow as a consequence of contamination with a winding molded bacterium found in the stomach called Helicobacter pylori (H. pylori). The microbes can likewise append to stomach cells, further debilitating the stomach's protective components. For reasons not totally comprehended, H. pylori can likewise empower the generation of acids in the stomach and cause tissue harm and irritation, which might at last result in a ulcer.

Stomach ulcer causes burning sensations in the mid-region behind the breastbone which can be particularly difficult when the stomach is vacant. Different side effects incorporate burping, queasiness, fatigue, acid reflux, regurgitating, midsection pain, dying, and loss of craving and weight.

Stomach settling agents and anti-microbiotics are utilized to treat such diseases., However, today microscopic organisms are developing progressively in imperviousness to anti-infection agents. Liquor, cigarettes, zesty foods, tea, and espresso are some gastric aggravations that ought to be stayed away from as they can conceivably irritate ulcer conditions. Taking a few little dinners for the duration of the day as opposed to eating three vast suppers can be useful as this means less acid generation in the stomach at every feast. A high fiber, low starch eating regimen, and vegetables, for example, cabbage and broccoli all advance ulcer recuperating. Additionally, drinking loads of water can ease ulcer issues.

The ulcerous condition, which is one or all the more moderate mending bruises, are frequently brought about by H-arch microscopic organisms. Your specialist can figure out whether this is the wellspring of your issue by leading analytic tests that may incorporate blood work and endoscopy, which is a tubal investigation of your stomach coating and throat. Some of the time, anxiety can assume a part in the improvement or exacerbation of ulcers. Check with your specialist about that and consider your way of life that may be having this harmful impact, and discover what you can do to enhance your every day routine and allay uneasiness from stomach ulcers.

Taking PeptoBismol or another acid neutralizer item before or after eating may diminish stomach corrosion and help reduce the severity of ulcers. Eating a few little suppers every day rather than a couple of substantial ones additionally may have influence in controlling the acid development that can prompt issues. Offset dinners containing fiery nourishments with those that are simpler on the stomach lining. Check with a nourishment expert or your specialist's office for proposals about the sustenance to avoid from and those you can eat to help control this condition.

The specialist may recommend a triple-treatment of anti-infection agents to demolish the microbes responsible for your ulcers. The course of treatment normally runs a few weeks, and a few patients need to take prescription for up to eight weeks. That ought to be the degree of the medication unless further issues are created.

You likewise can make moves to diminish stress from your life. Evade clashes with other individuals. Try not to be too hard on yourself. Keep a journal or individual diary for expounding on negative musings before they cause hurts. Getting normal activity for 30 minutes to an hour on most days is another awesome approach to decrease the impacts of anxiety and help you to stay sound. Your specialist can propose an activity that will fit with your way of life and general wellbeing.

Getting Having an ulcer is difficult thing, and it might be lengthy to get it under control. Look for notice signs like rectal dying, which may look like dark or delayed stools. Ceaseless acid reflux, trouble in gulping and perpetual burping may be pointers, too. Report any of these to your medicinal expert, and he or she will advice whether testing is expected to discount other conceivable reasons.

Natural remedies for Stomach Ulcers

If you have not understood, there are numerous characteristic solutions for treating stomach ulcers,. It is normal to get this excruciating condition these days. Common cures can generally be as compelling as the numerous pharmacological medications available, in most cases. Commonly, a bacterial stomach ulcer is dealt with by anti-infection agents. On the other hand, if your indications are gentle or if you wish to abstain from taking anti-infection agents, then you may wish to counsel your medicinal services supplier about utilizing some characteristic cures.

Around 80-90% of all instances of stomach ulcers are brought about by a microscopic organisms called Helicobacter Pylori. Stomach ulcers can likewise be brought about by a crumbling of the mucosal covering of the stomach that shields the stomach from corrosion . There are, additionally, different reasons for stomach ulcers. These include the secretion of excessive acidity, of, the abuse of meds, and smoking. Specialists additionally refer to hereditary inclination and push as variables that can bring about and trigger the advancement of ulcers. The utilization of specific meds, for example, an over the top utilization of headache medicine, can decline stomach ulcers.

Indications of stomach ulcers regularly appear like other complications. Thus, you may think that it's difficult to figure out whether you have them or not. The burning feeling in the upper mid-region brought about by stomach ulcers can be mistaken for acid reflux. The level of pain and the length of the pain changes with the person. Loss of hunger and weight reduction are likewise ordinarily experienced. Further side effects are heaving and bleeding stool.

if you are a smoker , or take excessive e ibuprofen or other ulcer triggering solutions, then you would need to guarantee that you eliminate the culpable substance by not making it your first step . At that point you can battle the ulcers with the accompanying regular cures:

• Herbs, for example, shoe elm and brilliant seal root can help lessen irritation and battle microscopic organisms.

• Add licorice to your eating regimen. It is a mitigating operators and it will help decrease stomach acid and bolster the stomach lining. Bite deglycyrrhizinated licorice before eating and at bed time.

- Eat bananas. This is a simple and normal approach to mitigate your stomach.

- Increase fiber in your eating regimen to keep the improvement of a few sorts of ulcers.

- Use vitamins that bolster the coating of your stomach, for example, Vitamin A and beta-carotene.

- Take 25 to 50 mg of zinc to help in mending.

- Look through your eating routine to figure out whether you ought to dispense with unfortunate dietary patterns. Unnecessary utilization of singed sustenance, for example, are bad for anybody. If you have stomach ulcers, you will need to remove conceivable compounding nourishments.

- Try unwinding strategies to diminish stress. A few tests show that the utilization of needle therapy, yoga, contemplation, and back rub helps the body to mend itself when you have ulcers.

Regular solutions for stomach ulcers are measures that you ought to check with your human services supplier, before leaving on them.

You ought not disregard the pain caused by stomach ulcers. It is vital to get to the base of your issue and discover approaches to battle it.

Ulcers and Gastrointestinal Bleeding

Draining in the GI tract is exceptionally basic. It ought not be disregarded in view of its potential genuine reasons and life debilitating results. Understanding fundamental terms and definitions utilized as a part of GI draining will make it less demanding for you to perceive GI draining in yourself or a relative, communicate all the more plainly to your specialist about your side effects, and scan all the more adequately and precisely for data. You will likewise be a more educated and viable backer for yourself so that the reason can be analyzed and treated precisely and in a convenient way.

Blood in the stool:

Blood in the stool or gastrointestinal tract may take different structures or appearances based on where it is originating from and how strong the problems is. There are basic restorative terms and definitions for blood in the gastrointestinal tract or stool that may not be commonplace to the lay but rather can be useful to know whether you or a relative has gastrointestinal complications. .

Hematemesis is spewing blood:

Red hematemesis is spewing red blood. Espresso ground's hematemesis is retching blood altered by stomach juices.

Blood in the stomach is truly sickening, normally bringing about retching. Retching blood is called hematemesis. It can be splendid red if happening quickly after the blood enters the stomach or when the draining is lively. Stomach acid and digestive juices modify any blood that remains in parts of the stomach. If the adjusted blood is regurgitated, it typically shows up like old espresso blend, henceforth the expression "coffee beans like" hematemesis. Blood may start from the stomach, be gulped, or spewed from the duodenum, the first piece of the small digestive tract soon after the stomach.

Melena and blood as an exceptionally strong purgative:

If blood in the stomach is not regurgitated totally, the modified blood goes into the digestive tract where it typically triggers looseness of the bowels. Then again, the looseness of the bowels is typically dark, dawdle and putrid. This is termed melena or melenic stool. Despite the fact that numerous specialists erroneously allude to such stool as melanotic, that is a mistaken term. "Melanotic" means containing melanin, the dim skin color present in moles and the threatening skin tumor, melanoma. Melena or melenic stools demonstrate an upper gastrointestinal tract drain or wellspring of blood in light of the fact that it has been adjusted by digestive juices present in the stomach and upper small digestive system. Such draining for the most part begins from a site reachable by an upper degree. However, once in a while the site is past the span of such a gastroscope.

Lower gastrointestinal drain and rectal degeneration:

Red blood passed through the rectum is an indication that the source of the flow is in the lower colon or rectum, or lower GI drain, with the exception of a monstrous discharge from the upper tract. Splendid red blood on bathroom tissue or trickling in the latrine dish is more often than not from the rear-end or rectum, most ordinarily from hemorrhoids or a butt-centric crevice, however it can also happen with a rectal disease.

Ulcers and Gastrointestinal Bleeding: Protecting Your Health

Draining in the GI tract is extremely basic. It ought not be overlooked in light of its potential genuine effects and life debilitating results. Understanding essential terms and definitions utilized as a part of GI draining will make it less demanding for you to perceive GI draining in yourself or a relative, communicate all the more obviously to your specialist about your side effects, and look all the more successfully and precisely for data. You will thus be a more informed and useful resource to yourself so that the reasons can be analyzed and treated precisely and in an auspicious way.

Blood in the stool:

Blood in the stool or gastrointestinal tract may take different structures or appearances based on where it is originating from and how real the situation is. . There are regular therapeutic terms and definitions for blood in the gastrointestinal tract or stool that may not be well known to the lay, but rather can be useful to know whether you or a relative has gastrointestinal issues.

Hematemesis is regurgitating blood:

Red hematemesis is regurgitating red blood. Espresso ground's hematemesis is spewing blood modified by stomach juices.

Blood in the stomach is very sickening because it brings about heaving. Spewing blood is called hematemesis. It can be splendid red if happening quickly after the blood enters the stomach or when the draining is lively. Stomach acid and digestive juices modify any blood that remains in parts of the stomach. If the adjusted blood is spewed, it generally shows up like old espresso blend, henceforth the expression "coffee blend like" hematemesis. Blood may start from the stomach, be gulped, or disgorged from the duodenum, the first piece of the small digestive tract soon after the stomach.

Melena and blood as an extremely intense purgative:

On the off chance that blood in the stomach is not spewed totally, the changed blood goes into the digestive system where it for the most part triggers looseness of the bowels. The resultant stuff is typically dark, dillydally and putrid. This is termed melena or melenic stool.. Melanotic alludes to containing melanin, the dim skin shade show in moles and the dangerous skin disease, melanoma. Melena or melenic stools demonstrate an upper gastrointestinal tract drain or wellspring of blood on the grounds that it has been modified by digestive squeezes just present in the stomach and upper small digestive system. Such draining for the most part starts from a site reachable by an upper extension, however, sometimes the site is past the compass of such a gastroscope.

Lower gastrointestinal discharge and rectal destruction:

Red blood passed rectally typically shows the wellspring of draining is in the lower colon or rectum, or lower GI drain, with the exception of in monstrous discharge from the upper tract. Splendid red blood on tissue or dribbling in the latrine dish is as a rule from the butt or rectum, most normally from hemorrhoids or a butt-centric gap, however can happen with rectal disease.

Ridiculous looseness of the bowels and colitis:

Ridiculous looseness of the bowels, frequently with bodily fluid, is common in colitis. Colitis is aggravation of the colon or digestive organs from any of various reasons that may include contamination, poor blood stream to the digestive tract (ischemia) and the constant incendiary entrail maladies, ulcerative colitis and Crohn's infection.

Mysterious blood in the stool:

It takes around 50-100 ml of blood to turn the stool dark or melenic. Under 2 measures of draining is in this manner not for the most part obviously noticeable and is termed mysterious blood in the stool. Different compound tests for mysterious blood in the stool exist that should be possible on emptied stool or stool obtained by a gloved finger for examination by a specialist. Mysterious blood in the stool is enough concern for disease and it requires an assessment for that reason. Ulcers, indigestion, Celiac illness, polyps, colitis and Crohn's infection, hemorrhoids and headache medicines cause damage to the gastrointestinal tract and are all normal non-disease reasons for mysterious blood in the stool.

Stomach Ulcer treatment

Stomach ulcer treatment for the most part can be achieved through three different techniques. Any of these three sorts can be connected exclusively, yet there are cases in which each one of them can be connected all the while, particularly when the manifestations are serious. and have created a way for confusions like draining and puncturing.

- Acid-stifling drugs. This sort of stomach ulcer treatment utilized a specific class of medications that you ought to take for four to eight weeks. Its primary intention is to greatly reduce the amount of acids delivered by the stomach. This class of medications takes a shot at the defensive cells of the stomach's coating and ulcers generally recuperate as the measure of acids diminishes altogether.

- Clearing of helicobacter pylori. Typically, as already stated, most stomach ulcer cases are brought about by helicobacter pylori contamination. Consequently, the real concern of the stomach ulcer treatment is the entry point of the helicobacter disease. It is a reality that acid smothering pharmaceuticals alone are insufficient for the treatment of stomach ulcers. The contamination ought to be completely eradicated to avoid from a repeat of the illness. Anti-infection agents are utilized to clear the contamination. Acid smothering medication is expected to make anti-toxins stronger.. It likewise serves to decrease the acids created in the stomach.

The pathway of the contamination will diminish the conceivable repeat of the ulcer.

● Avoiding the ongoing utilization of calming medications. A mitigating medication may contribute to the creation of acids in the stomach. Maintaining a strategic distance from the ongoing utilization of mitigating medications will permit ulcers in the stomach to recuperate and the possibility of it occurring again will be decreased. Some of the time, a person who experiences joint pain or other agonizing conditions may take mitigating medication to recuperate the swelling of the joints. Matching the calming medications with acid suppressants is likely to be able to counteract ulcers, which could otherwise add to the excruciating condition. In terms of taking medications, it is better to talk about it with your specialist for counsel on the most proficient method to counter the symptoms associated with the medications.

To avoid from the intricacies concerning ulcers or to completely treat ulcers in the stomach, one of the first things you must do is to alter your way of life.

CONCLUSION

You may find yourself looking into the mirror and the first thing you may notice is a fat stomach. This happens to numerous individuals and is commonly an ordinary aftereffect of carrying on with your life. You might as well see that your lower stomach is the territory that stands out the most and that which leaves you with the ugliest memory. Stomach fat begins to assemble at the least purpose of gravity, which is your lower stomach. It hangs off of your body in an exceptionally ugly way, and it will keep on gathering and in the end assemble fat upon fat and in this manner make your entire stomach stand out and look awful.

All right, because your lower stomach the primary spot fat begins to develop, it is the last place that you will lose fat. So, if you truly need to lose the additional fat that hangs on your lower stomach, you have to lose whatever is left of your stomach fat first. It would be decent if there were an easy route, but there isn't. Stomach fat is based at your midsection and it begins at your lower stomach and simply exacerbated from that point. So if stomach fat is the issue, where do activities come in? All things considered, exercises won't have the capacity to burn off the majority of the essential fat without anyone else's input. However, it can fortify the muscles underneath the fat so as to give it a superior capacity of supporting the weight and keeping your stomach from sagging significantly.

www.ingramcontent.com/pod-product-compliance
Lightning Source LLC
Chambersburg PA
CBHW051904170526
45168CB00001B/236